PRENTICE-HALL
FOUNDATIONS OF IMMUNOLOGY SERIES

EDITORS

Abraham G. Osler

*The Public Health Research Institute of the City of New York
and New York University School of Medicine*

Leon Weiss

The Johns Hopkins University School of Medicine

RADIOIMMUNOASSAY

OF

BIOLOGICALLY ACTIVE COMPOUNDS

CHARLES W. PARKER

Washington University School of Medicine

PRENTICE-HALL, INC., *Englewood Cliffs, New Jersey*

Library of Congress Cataloging in Publication Data

PARKER, CHARLES WARD, (date)
Radioimmunoassay of biologically active compounds.

(Foundations of immunology series)
Bibliography: p.
Includes index.
1. Radioimmunoassay. I. Title. [DNLM: 1. Radio-
immunoassay. QY250 P238r]
QR188.5.P37   616.07′9′028   76-4987
ISBN 0-13-750505-1

QR188.5
P37

10   9   8   7   6   5   4   3   2   1

PRINTED IN THE UNITED STATES OF AMERICA

PRENTICE-HALL INTERNATIONAL, INC., *London*
PRENTICE-HALL OF AUSTRALIA PTY. LIMITED, *Sydney*
PRENTICE-HALL OF CANADA, LTD., *Toronto*
PRENTICE-HALL OF INDIA PRIVATE LIMITED, *New Delhi*
PRENTICE-HALL OF JAPAN, INC., *Tokyo*
PRENTICE-HALL OF SOUTHEAST ASIA PTE., LTD., *Singapore*

To my parents, William B. Parker and Florence M. Parker,
for their continued encouragement and love.

Foundations of Immunology Series

This series of monographs is intended to provide readers of diverse backgrounds with an authoritative and clear statement concerning significant aspects of immunology. Each volume represents an individual contribution by a distinguished scientist. As a series, they provide a comprehensive view of the field.

The editors have encouraged the individuality of each author in content and method of presentation. They have sought as the major objective of the series, that each monograph be comprehensible and of interest to a broad audience. The authors provide an authoritative treatment of important problems in major research areas, in which rapid development of new information requires an integrated and reliable evaluation. The series should therefore prove valuable to advanced college students, graduate students, medical students and house staff, practitioners of medicine, laboratory scientists, and teachers.

ABRAHAM G. OSLER
LEON WEISS

Contents

Preface

My interest in immunoassays dates back to 1960 when I was a fellow in Dr. Herman Eisen's laboratory and my wife, Dr. Mary Parker, and her colleagues, Dr. William Daughaday and Dr. Robert Utiger, were working to develop a radioimmunoassay for human growth hormone. At that time very few people including myself fully appreciated the enormous impact that sensitive immunological methods would have both in scientific investigation and in the performance of routine clinical measurements. Barring unforeseen technological developments, the present rapid rate of growth in the immunoassay field will no doubt continue for at least another decade. Despite the large number of immunoassays that have already been generated and implemented, the development and intelligent utilization of new assays is subject to many pitfalls particularly if the investigator does not have a clear understanding of the fundamental principle of immunological reactivity and specificity laid down by the work of Landsteiner, Avery, Heidelburger, Eisen, Campbell, Pressman, Kabat, and Karush, among many others. While the general subject of immunoassays has been reviewed repeatedly, there have been few attempts to provide practical information on immunoassay methodology alongside a detailed discussion of what it is that makes a substance antigenic, how antibodies are optimally prepared and evaluated, and the general nature of the interaction of an antibody with an antigen in terms of binding specificity and cross-reactivity and the kinetics and thermodynamics of antigen-antibody interactions. The desirability of providing this information to non-immunologists who wish to utilize immunoassays has become increasingly apparent from informal discussions with colleagues and co-investigators at Washington University School of Medicine over a period of many years. Thus this book is written more for pharmacologists, biochemists, physiologists and cellular biologists than it is for immunologists. Obviously the vast literature dealing with immunoassays could not be covered comprehensively in a monograph of this size, and where illustrations are used no doubt examples exist in other immunoassay systems which would have been equally appropriate.

I am indebted to my colleagues for helpful criticisms, particularly my wife, Dr. Mary Parker, and to Mrs. Evelyn Oberbeck and Mrs. Deborah Noakes for their help with the manuscript. I am also grateful to the National Institute of Allergy and Infectious Diseases which provided the research and career development support involved in my own work in the immunoassay field.

CHARLES W. PARKER

Chapter 1

Introduction

Historically, radioiodinated antigens and antibodies were first used by immunologists in the study of antigen-antibody reactions (Pressman and Eisen, 1950). Within a short time the use of radiolabeled proteins was extended to studies of the in vivo metabolism of proteins (Berson et al., 1953). This work led to the demonstration of circulating anti-insulin antibodies in individuals being treated with foreign insulins (Berson et al., 1956). Berson and Yalow (1958) were the first to point out the remarkable sensitivity possible when unlabeled antigens are measured by their ability to inhibit competitively the binding of highly radiolabeled antigens by antibody. Subsequent to their initial description, radioimmunoassays were rapidly developed for other protein and polypeptide hormones (Unger et al., 1959; Grodsky and Forsham, 1960; Utiger et al., 1962). Our laboratory extended the radioimmunoassay concept to small molecular weight drugs that must be coupled to proteins in order to produce antibodies (Oliver et al., 1966; Oliver et al., 1968; Steiner et al., 1969; Spector and Parker, 1970; Jaffe et al., 1971; Parker, 1974). During the past 10 years radioimmunoassays have emerged as an important tool in biologic research. Knowledge in such diverse areas as endocrinology (the protein and polypeptide hormones), cellular biology (cyclic AMP and cyclic GMP), and pharmacology (digitalis, morphine) has been greatly expanded by the application of this technique.

Most radioimmunoassays use radioiodinated antigens and depend on the ability of unlabeled antigen (Ag) to inhibit the binding of labeled antigen (Ag*) when limited amounts of specific antibody (Ab) are present. This process may be viewed as a simple competition in which Ag reduces the amount of free Ab, thus decreasing the availability of Ab to Ag*:

$$(1) \qquad Ag \cdot Ab \; \rightleftarrows \; Ag + Ab + Ag^* \; \rightleftarrows \; Ag^* \cdot Ab$$

In performing the assay, Ag* and Ab are incubated in the presence and absence of samples containing Ag. After reaching or approaching equilibrium, free Ag* and antibody-bound Ag* are separated and one or the

1

other is determined by radioactive counting. The antigen concentration in the unknown is measured by comparing the diminution of Ag* binding produced by Ag in the sample to that of a standard curve obtained by adding graded, known amounts of Ag to the assay system (Fig. 1.1).

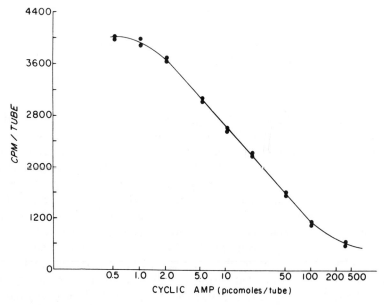

Fig. 1.1. Typical standard immunoassay curve for cyclic AMP. Each tube contained 0.1 pmole ^{125}I-SCAMP-TME (succinyl-cAMP-tyrosine methyl ester labeled with ^{125}I) and a final anticyclic AMP-antibody dilution of 1:2,000. (Taken from A. L. Steiner, D. M. Kipnis, R. Utiger, and C. Parker. 1969. Proc. Nat. Acad. Sci. USA. 64:367–373.)

Since what is measured in radioimmunoassays is the ability of the unknown to produce a competitive change in the binding of antigen by antibody, any quantitative method for studying antigen-antibody reactions can be utilized in principle. In the past few years a number of variations have been described: (a) Radiolabeled antibodies or nonradioactive markers for either antigen or antibody have been used to follow the reaction. (b) Naturally occurring tissue- or serum-binding proteins with affinity for the unknown have been used as substitutes for antibody. Eventually synthetic polymers or proteins might be employed for the same purpose, provided that they can be constructed so as to provide the necessary level of binding specificity. (c) Methods have also been developed in which bound antigen can be measured in the presence of free antigen, thereby obviating the need to separate free and bound antigen. In principle, it does not matter whether it is the antigen or the antibody that is labeled nor how the measurement is made as long as the binding is specific, there is adequate discrimination between the free and bound species, and the required sensitivity is obtained.

The current widespread application of immunoassays is not difficult to understand. With an antibody of high affinity for antigen and a label on the antigen or antibody of high specific activity, picogram quantities of antigen can be measured. Few, if any, other assay procedures provide the combination of sensitivity, specificity, versatility, and convenience that immunoassays offer. But like other quantitative methods, immunoassays can present serious problems in development or can be misused, thus yielding inadequate or misleading information. The development and optimal utilization of highly sensitive immunoassays require the appropriate application of a number of simple but important immunochemical principles. This monograph is concerned with those principles as well as with current and possible future developments in immunoassay technology.

Chapter 2

Immunogens

CLASSES OF IMMUNOGENS

The word *immunogen* has come to refer to any substance that, under suitable conditions, can induce antibody formation. In order for a substance to have this capability, it must be part of a macromolecule. Although it has long been known that proteins stimulate antibody formation, it is now recognized that carbohydrates, lipopolysaccharides, nucleic acids, and even relatively small polypeptides may serve as antibody inducers. Sizable proteins (molecular weights in excess of 10,000 daltons) are particularly potent immunogens, provided that they are foreign to the immunized animal (e.g., from a species that is sufficiently different phylogenetically). The experience in obtaining antibodies to polypeptides in the 1,000 to 10,000 molecular weight size is much more variable, with some polypeptides readily eliciting antibody formation and others exhibiting little if any immunogenicity, even when given repeatedly in adjuvant (Parker, 1971). Bovine and porcine insulin are relatively potent immunogens. Glucagon, ACTH, calcitonin, and gastrin, as unconjugated polypeptides, have produced an immune response when given repeatedly in complete adjuvant, but by ordinary standards they are weak immunogens. Even oxytocin, which has only eight amino acids, is capable of inducing an immune response (Gilliland and Prout, 1965), but it should be noted that the oxytocin contains an amide group that might conceivably promote conjugation to protein in vivo. Some peptides—angiotensin II, for example—that fail to elicit antibody production when administered in adjuvant may do so when the peptide is absorbed to a solid particle, such as carbon black (Boyd and Peart, 1968), or a plastic bead.

Factors in the relatively low immunogenicity of small polypeptides probably include rapid excretion or destruction and lack of immunological complexity. Most small polypeptides are rapidly filtered into the tubular urine at the glomerulus, and some are so susceptible to proteolysis by enzymes present in blood tissue that their half lives in the circulation

4

are only a few minutes. In addition, several of the more immunogenic, small molecular weight polypeptides have a greater tendency to polymerize than the less-immunogenic polypeptides. Bovine insulin, for example, has a molecular weight of only about 6,000 daltons but may contain aggregates as large as 48,000 daltons. When the higher molecular weight aggregates are eliminated, the immunogenicity of insulin is considerably reduced (Root et al., 1972). Even with polypeptides that are less prone to aggregate, the water-in-oil emulsions that are used as vehicles in immunization might be expected to promote association between polypeptide molecules at the water-oil interface. Indeed, some of the larger molecules, such as bovine serum albumin (molecular weight 70,000), may also have to be aggregated in order to express their full immunogenicity. In several animal species, ultracentrifuged, monomeric preparations of serum albumin or gamma globulin are poorly immunogenic, or even tolerogenic, unless they are given in adjuvant, which partially restores the response (Dresser, 1962; Frei et al., 1965).

Because of the uncertainty that a small polypeptide will produce an effective response, the question arises as to whether to immunize with an emulsion of the free polypeptide or with a conjugate of the polypeptide to a protein. As a rule, it is much easier to obtain a significant antibody response if the polypeptide is attached to a protein carrier. Conjugation not only reduces the need for frequent injections of polypeptide and the total quantity of antigen necessary for immunization but is also more likely to provide suitable antisera after immunization of limited numbers of animals. Most investigators who initially utilized unconjugated polypeptides for immunization subsequently elected to immunize exclusively with polypeptides conjugated to protein. Orth, for example, had to immunize more than 200 guinea pigs with unconjugated ACTH in order to obtain a single useful antiserum (Orth, 1974). Much more consistent results were obtained by immunization with α^{1-24} ACTH conjugated to bovine serum albumin. Less strikingly, Jaffe and Walsh (1974) observed that only 3 out of 14 rabbits immunized with crude porcine gastin produced antibodies, whereas every one of a number of rabbits immunized with gastin conjugated to albumin developed antibodies suitable for radioimmunoassay use.

Theoretically, for small polypeptide molecules that are produced in vivo by proteolysis from larger protein precursors, immunization with the precursor might be effective. This situation has been demonstrated in the bradykinin-bradykininogen system by Pierce and Webster (1966). However, it is doubtful that the approach is generally applicable, because of the possibility that other areas of the protein molecule would dominate the immune response.

Under ordinary circumstances drugs and intracellular metabolites with molecular weights of below 1,000 are not immunogenic at all unless they are attached to an immunogenic carrier, such as a protein (Landsteiner, 1936; Eisen, 1959; Parker, 1965a). The term *hapten* is used to describe a nonimmunogenic molecule that acquires immunogenicity after attachment to a carrier, and therefore it includes nonimmunogenic oligopeptides, lipids, sugars, and polynucleotides as well as drugs. It would appear that antibodies can be produced to an unlimited variety of organic molecules, including important endogenous metabolites that are widely distributed in animal tissues. In order to immunize with a hapten, it is necessary that the bond between the hapten and the protein be relatively stable. Thus small organic molecules bound to proteins either through covalent or coordination linkages can initiate an immune response, but there is no indication that more readily reversible bonds of the type that these agents form with serum albumins and other proteins can do so (Parker, 1972a). To be sure, electrostatic complexes between immunogenic proteins and DNA can give rise to anti-DNA antibodies, whereas uncomplexed DNA is ordinarily a poor immunogen (Plescia et al., 1964). This is a special situation in which long, oppositely charged polypeptide and polynucleotide chains create an opportunity for the summation of ionic binding energies and the formation of a very stable complex. Thus the promotion of an antihapten response depends on the overall stability of the hapten-protein complex rather than on any special chemical properties of the bonds themselves.

The effectiveness of hapten-protein conjugates as immunogens does not completely rule out the possibility that unconjugated haptens might initiate an immune response (Parker, 1972a) under special circumstances. *p*-Azobenzenearsonates and 2,4-dinitrophenyl (DNP) amino acids that are unattached to proteins have been reported to induce allergic skin responses in vivo (Leskowitz et al., 1966; Frey et al., 1969), particularly when administered in complete adjuvant, whereas DNP amino acids also stimulate DNA synthesis in bone marrow cells from unimmunized rabbits in vitro (Eisen et al., 1971). The immune response to benzenearsonate has special features in that delayed hypersensitivity is induced in the apparent absence of a detectable serum antibody response (Leskowitz et al., 1966). The difficulty in interpretation comes from the possibility that the unconjugated hapten might contain impurities or be immunogenic only after metabolic processing that leads to the formation of protein-bound derivatives (Parker, 1965b). If the structural alteration leading to immunogenicity were great enough, the antibodies obtained might not cross-react immunologically with the original benzenearsonate molecule and so would remain undetected. Using DNP amino acids, Frey and his colleagues have attempted to distinguish between direct immunogenicity and contamination or metabolic processing of the hapten (Frey et al., 1969). They found that different preparations of the same, apparently pure DNP amino acid varied markedly in their capacity to produce delayed hypersensitivity. They raised the possibility that low, ordinarily undetectable levels of contamination of certain DNP-amino acid preparations with protein-reactive impurities might explain this variation. Although further investigation is warranted, present evidence is support of direct immunization by unconjugated haptens is unconvincing; even if unequivocal evidence for direct immunization is eventually obtained, the use of hapten-protein conjugates would presumably still be preferable in preparing high-affinity antibodies for immunoassay purposes.

CONSIDERATIONS IN PREPARING HAPTEN-PROTEIN CONJUGATES FOR IMMUNIZATION

Types of Coupling Reagents

Most small molecules of biologic interest do not have intrinsic protein reactivity, and, in order to obtain a stable bond with a protein, an activating agent is necessary. Three classes of agents are commonly used: (a) those that form a bridge between amino groups (diisocyanates, diimido esters, dihalonitrobenzenes, glutaldehyde); (b) those that bridge between tyrosyl, histidyl, or lysyl residues (bifunctional diazonium salts); and (c) those that activate carboxyl groups (usually on the hapten) so that they react with amino groups (usually on the protein), thus forming a CO—NH bond (carbodiimides, alkyl chloroformates, and isoxazolium salts). Many of the carboxylate activating agents are the same ones that are used in the synthesis of peptides and oligonucleotides. Formulas for these reactions and a summary of the conditions under which they are used are given in Fig. 2.1 and Table 2.1. A number of different types of conjugation procedures are illustrated in Williams and Chase (1967).

Choosing a Conjugation Procedure

The choice of a conjugation procedure is influenced by the stability and solubility properties of the hapten, the groups on the hapten available for conjugation, the particular mode of attachment to the protein that is desired, and, to a certain extent, by pragmatism. When we began preparing conjugates of prostaglandins with proteins some years ago, the possibility of altering the labile cyclopentane ring of PGE_1 with conversion to other prostaglandins during conjugation had to be considered, and for this reason conjugation by means of a mixed anhydride appeared preferable to a carbodiimide-mediated conjugation. When antibodies obtained with the two conjugates were compared, this predication turned out to be accurate. Useful anti-PGE_1 antibodies were obtained only after immunization with the mixed anhydride conjugate (Jaffe et al., 1973; Jaffe

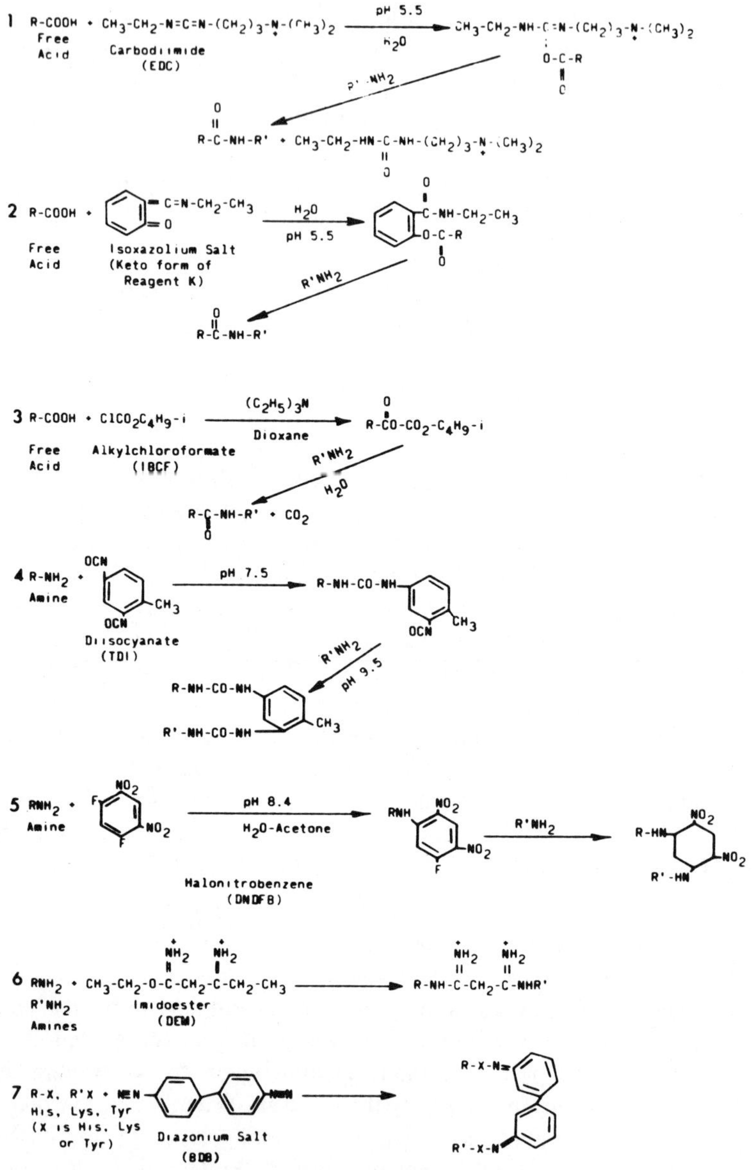

1 R-COOH + CH$_3$-CH$_2$-N=C=N-(CH$_2$)$_3$-N-(CH$_3$)$_2$ $\xrightarrow[\text{H}_2\text{O}]{\text{pH 5.5}}$ CH$_3$-CH$_2$-NH-C=N-(CH$_2$)$_3$-N-(CH$_3$)$_2$
   Free   Carbodiimide   O-C-R
   Acid   (EDC)   ‖
                                                                                              O

   R'-NH$_2$

   O
   ‖
   R-C-NH-R' + CH$_3$-CH$_2$-HN-C-NH-(CH$_2$)$_3$-N-(CH$_3$)$_2$
                                ‖
                                O

2 R-COOH + [benzene ring]—C=N-CH$_2$-CH$_3$ $\xrightarrow[\text{pH 5.5}]{\text{H}_2\text{O}}$ [benzene ring with] O
                            =O   ‖
   Free   Isoxazolium Salt   -NH-CH$_2$-CH$_3$
   Acid   (Keto form of   -O-C-R
             Reagent K)   ‖
                                                                                              O
                          R'-NH$_2$

   O
   ‖
   R-C-NH-R'

3 R-COOH + ClCO$_2$C$_4$H$_9$-i $\xrightarrow[\text{Dioxane}]{(C_2H_5)_3N}$ R-CO-CO$_2$-C$_4$H$_9$-i
   Free   Alkylchloroformate
   Acid   (IBCF)   R'-NH$_2$
                                       H$_2$O

   R-C-NH-R' + CO$_2$
     ‖
     O

4 R-NH$_2$ + [benzene ring with OCN, OCN, CH$_3$] $\xrightarrow{\text{pH 7.5}}$ R-NH-CO-NH-[benzene ring with OCN, CH$_3$]
   Amine   Diisocyanate
              (TDI)
                                                    R'-NH$_2$
                                                    pH 9.5

   R-NH-CO-NH-[benzene ring]
                        CH$_3$
   R'-NH-CO-NH

5 RNH$_2$ + [benzene ring with NO$_2$, F, NO$_2$] $\xrightarrow[\text{H}_2\text{O-Acetone}]{\text{pH 8.4}}$ RNH-[benzene ring with NO$_2$, F, NO$_2$] $\xrightarrow{\text{R'-NH}_2}$ R-HN-[ring with NO$_2$, NO$_2$]-R'-HN
   Amine   Malonitrobenzene
             (DNDFB)

6 RNH$_2$ + CH$_3$-CH$_2$-O-C-CH$_2$-C-CH$_2$-CH$_3$ $\longrightarrow$ R-NH-C-CH$_2$-C-NHR'
   R'NH$_2$ ‖NH$_2$ ‖NH$_2$ ‖NH$_2$ ‖NH$_2$
   Amines   Imidoester
              (DEM)

7 R-X, R'X + N≡N-[biphenyl]-N≡N $\longrightarrow$ R-X-N=[ring]
   His, Lys, Tyr
   (X is His, Lys   R'-X-N=[ring]
    or Tyr)   Diazonium Salt
                (BDB)

Fig. 2.1. Reactions used in the conjugation of haptens to proteins. R'-NH$_2$ is a protein HN$_2$ group and R is the hapten. (Taken from C. W. Parker. 1971. *In* W. D. Odell, and W. H. Daughaday (Eds.). Principles of competitive protein-binding assays. J. B. Lippincott Co., Philadelphia, pp. 25–48.)

Table 2.1

Reagents for the conjugation of haptens to protein. EDC, 1-ethyl-3-(3-dimethyl-aminopropyl) carbodiimide. HCL; CMC,1-cyclohexyl-3-(2-morpholinyl-4-ethyl) carbodiimide methyl p-toluene sulfonate; DCC, N,N'-dicyclohexylcarbodiimide; reagent K, N-ethyl-5-phenylisoxazolium-3'-sulfonate; ECF, ethylchloroformate; IBCF, isobutylchloroformate; TDI, toluene 2,4-diisocyanate; XDI, xylylenediisocyanate; DNDFB, 2,4-dinitro-1,5-difluorobenzene; FNPS, p,p'-difluoro-, m,m'-dinitrodiphenylsulfone; DEM, diethyl malonimidate; BDB, bisdiazotized benzidine. (Taken from Parker, 1971.)

Coupling agent	Reaction steps	Coupling Agents Water solubility	Coupling Agents Optimal pH	Solvent	Bond formed
1. Carbodiimides					
a. EDC	1 or 2	high	5.5	H_2O	CO—NH
b. CMC	1 or 2	high	5.5	H_2O	CO—NH
c. DCC	1 or 2	low	–	nonaqueous	CO—NH
2. Isoxazolium					
Salts	1 or 2	high	5.5	H_2O	CO—NH
Reagent K					
3. Alkylchloroformates	2	low	(1)-	dioxane	CO—NH
ECF, IBCF			(2)9.0	dioxane-H_2O	
4. Diisocyanates	2	low	(1)7.5	H_2O	NH—R—NH
TDI, XDI			(2)9.5	H_2O	
5. Halonitrobenzenes					
a. DNDFB	1 or 2	low	8.5	acetone-H_2O	NH—R—NH
b. FNPS	1	low	10.0		
6. Imidoesters					
DEM	1	high	9.0	H_2O	NH^+—R^+—NH
7. Diazonium					
Salts	1	high	7.5	H_2O	X—R—X
BDB					(X = His, Tyr, Lys)

and Behrman, 1974). Another consideration is the linkage that is desired. As discussed in greater detail below, antibodies tend to be specific for the portion of the hapten most distal to the point of attachment to protein (Parker, 1971). Ideally, attachment should take place in the area of the hapten that is least important for immunological recognition. This prin-

PGE   PGA   PGB   PGF

ciple was utilized by Haber (1969) in the development of immunoassays for angiotensin I, a decapeptide, and angiotensin II, an octapeptide formed from angiotensin I by cleavage of the two C-terminal amino acids (Fig. 2.2). In studies of angiotensin metabolism, it is sometimes necessary to be

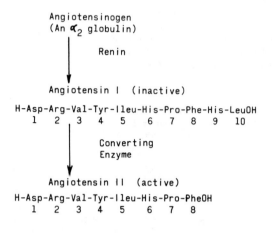

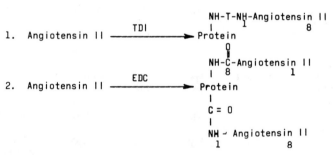

Fig. 2.2. Possible methods of conjugation of angiotensin II to protein. TDI is toluene diisocyanate; EDC is a water-soluble carbodiimide (see Fig. 2.1 and Table 2.1). (Taken from C. W. Parker. 1971. *In* W. D. Odell, and W. H. Daughaday (Eds.) Principles of competitive protein-binding assays. J.B. Lippincott Co., Philadelphia. pp. 25–48.)

able to distinguish between the two peptides. Immunological differentiation is possible with antibodies to conjugates in which the polypeptide is coupled through the N-terminal portion of the molecule. With antibodies to angiotensin I-toluene diisocyanate-protein conjugates (attachment largely or entirely through the N-terminal amino group), cross-reactivity with angiotensin II was only about 2%. Antibodies to angiotensin II, also coupled through the N-terminal end, cross-reacted with angiotensin I to the extent of about 5%. When antibodies to polypeptides attached through the opposite end of the molecule were used, little or no difference in binding was obtained because immunological recognition was primarily directed toward identical regions of the two polypeptides.

Selective conjugation reactions may also be desirable with intermediate-sized polypeptides that have considerable tertiary structure and depend on specified functional amino acid residues to maintain this structure in solution. In this situation, it may be advantageous to use a bifunctional imidoester; bifunctional imidoesters not only are selective for amino groups but also replace a positive charge for every ϵ-ammonium group that is substituted. As discussed below, proteins and polypeptides that are reacted with imidoesters show little or no alteration in average charge, optical rotation, and viscosity. Bifunctional imidoesters have been used advantageously in the preparation of antibodies to glucagon (Grey et al., 1970). Since glucagon has only two amino groups available for conjugation in the entire polypeptide (at the α-amino position and the single lysyl residue at position 13), the reaction is a relatively selective one, considering the size of the polypeptide (29 amino acids).

Regardless of the conjugation procedure used, exposure of the protein to the coupling agent will result in cross linking of functional groups on different protein molecules and aggregation. Extensively cross-linked proteins often have reduced solubility. This feature is not necessarily disadvantageous, since partially insolubilized proteins often are effective immunogens. Haptenic groups can sometimes be activated in the absence of protein, unreacted activating agent removed, and conjugation to protein carried out with little or no risk of cross linking of protein molecules. Toluene diisocyanate and dinitrodifluorobenzene (Fig. 2.1) are examples of reagents in which the initial reaction products are sufficiently stable to permit two-step reactions. If the hapten contains free carboxylate groups, it can often be converted to an acid chloride or active ester, both of which have intrinsic protein reactivity. Sugars with vicinal hydroxyl groups can be coupled directly to protein following oxidation with periodate, thereby leading to the formation (Fig. 2.3) of a dialdehyde (Erlanger, 1973). After the aldehyde groups have been allowed to combine directly with protein amino groups, thus forming a Schiff's base-type linkage, the attachment is stabilized by reduction with sodium borohydride.

In addition to their action in promoting peptide bond formation, carbodiimides can be used to conjugate mononucleotides and oligonucleotides to protein (Halloran and Parker, 1964, 1966). A phosphoamide bond is formed through 3′ or 5′ phosphate groups on the nucleotide and amino groups on the protein (Fig. 2.4). This method has been utilized to prepare antibodies to a variety of ribo- and deoxyribonucleotides, including DNA (Halloran and Parker, 1966) and tRNA (Bonavida et al., 1970), and should be applicable to any nucleotide containing free phosphate groups. Nucleoside conjugation can also be accomplished by the direct

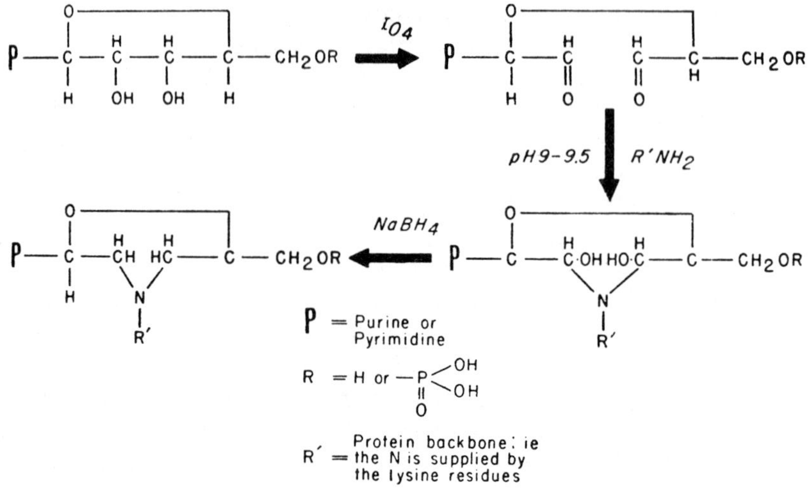

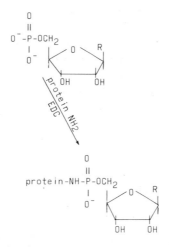

Fig. 2.3. The periodate method of preparing nucleoside- or nucleotide-protein conjugates. (Taken from B. F. Erlanger, and S. M. Beiser. 1964. Proc. Nat. Acad. Sci. USA. 52:68–74.)

Fig. 2.4. Conjugation of a nucleotide to a protein using a water-soluble carbodiimide. Modified from Halloran and Parker (1966).

reaction of trichloromethyl nucleosides, with proteins (Butler et al., 1962). With ribonucleotides, conjugation can occur by periodate oxidation as described above. A frequently used reaction for attaching sugars or steroids to proteins involves the formation of esters or ethers containing *p*-nitrophenyl groups (Landsteiner, 1936). After reduction, the *p*-nitrophenyl group is converted to an aromatic amine. The amine is diazotized and attached to protein through an azo linkage (Fig. 2.5).

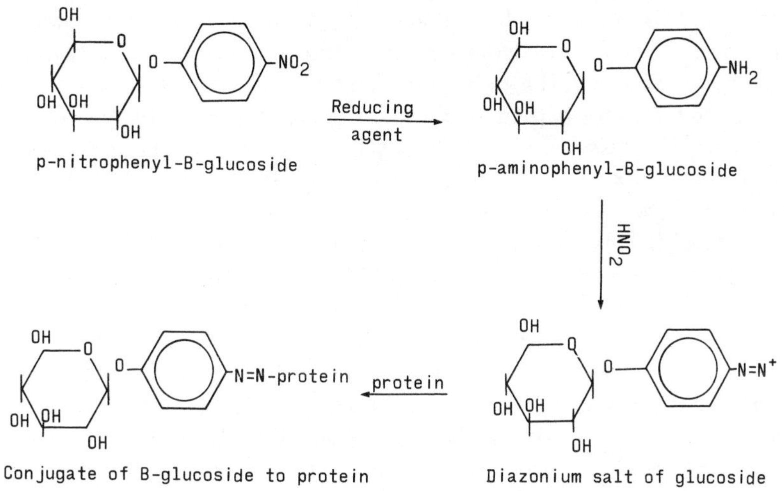

Fig. 2.5. Conjugation of a monosaccharide to a protein through formation of the *p*-nitrophenyl ester, reduction, and diazotization.

Most or all of the commonly used coupling agents participate in side reactions with protein and induce the formation of self-directed antibodies. For example, the water-soluble carbodiimide, EDC, is capable of reacting covalently with protein amino groups, thus creating a guanidino substituent that is immunogenic in its own right (Goodfriend et al., 1964). If the possibility of antibodies to the coupling agent is not considered, problems in interpretation will arise if the antiserum is analyzed for precipitating antibodies by using a hapten-protein conjugate prepared with the same coupling agent. As discussed elsewhere, other side reactions that occur during conjugation of haptens to protein include the cross linking of protein molecules, structural rearrangements of the hapten or denaturation associated with exposure of the protein to organic solvents, protein-precipitating reagents, or extremes of pH (see below).

Conditions for Conjugation

Since most of the conjugation reactions are bimolecular in character, conjugation is generally carried out at relatively high concentrations of protein and hapten with continuous stirring to increase the likelihood of binding of hapten to the protein. When the hapten is relatively insoluble in aqueous solution, the addition of 5 to 25% by volume of an inert inorganic solvent may be considered in an effort to improve the conjugation efficiency. Once the reaction is completed, the protein is purified by extensive dialysis or chromatography in order to remove unreacted hapten and is analyzed for attached haptenic groups. If available, a radioactive hapten is used during conjugation to facilitate the analysis of conjugation efficiency. If a radioactive hapten is not available, any quantitative method for the hapten that has the needed sensitivity and that can be used in the presence of protein may be considered. If the hapten-amino acid linkage is stable to acid hydrolysis, the protein may be degraded to its constituent amino acids and analysed. Analysis by subtraction (by determination of unsubstituted functional amino acid residues before and after conjugation) can also be attempted but may give falsely high values because of functional group involvement in side reactions with the coupling agent. Regardless of the analytical procedure used, the possibility of degradation or rearrangement of the hapten during conjugation must be considered. In this connection, it should be noted that ordinarily radioactive measurements will not reveal changes in hapten structure, whereas spectrophotometric or fluorometric measurements may or may not do so.

Serious problems in interpretation can occur if the hapten is hydrophobic, thereby leading to inefficient removal by dialysis and a falsely high estimate of covalent hapten substitution. It may be necessary to dialyse for periods of up to 7 to 10 days with regular changes of the dialysate to ensure that the removal of noncovalently bound hapten is nearing completion. If the protein does not denature readily, it can be extracted with an organic solvent, such as 95% ethanol or acetone, at low temperature to obviate this problem.

Desirable Levels of Substitution

In the past it was considered desirable to substitute the protein as heavily as possible with hapten; consequently, relatively high molar ratios of hapten and coupling agent to protein have been used (e.g., a five- to one hundredfold molar excess of hapten over reactive amino acid residues on the protein). Glutaraldehyde conjugation procedures have been an exception in that it is more usual to match the number of hapten and protein amino groups. Satisfactory responses to immunization have been achieved with 3'O-carboxymethylmorphine, 2'O-succinyl-cyclic AMP, and prostaglandin-protein conjugates containing an average of only two to six haptenic groups per protein molecule (Spector and Parker, 1970; Steiner et al., 1969; Jaffe et al., 1971). Indeed, studies with mono-DNP derivatives of ribonuclease (Eisen et al., 1964), insulin (Little and Counts, 1969), and oligolysine indicate that a single haptenic group per molecule of carrier is sufficient to produce antihapten antibody. The success in immunizing with monovalent DNP preparations may seem surprising, for it is widely assumed that a multivalent interaction is needed in order to perturb the lymphocyte surface sufficiently to produce cell activation (Rajewsky et al., 1969) (see below). Presumably a multivalent interaction is indeed required, but either the immunogen is undergoing aggregation in vivo or all but one of the valences can be provided by the protein or oligopeptide carrier, possibly in combination with the surface of a contiguous cell. Not only are high levels of hapten substitution unnecessary for immunization, but it is conceivable that they are undesirable as well. According to present-day concepts of immunological induction, conjugates with a low multiplicity of haptenic groups are less apt to trigger cells with a low affinity for hapten than conjugates with larger numbers of haptenic groups. A study suggesting that high levels of substitution may actually be detrimental was reported by Tigelaar et al. (1973). They conjugated diphenylhydantoin to protein, separating a relatively lightly substituted, soluble protein fraction from a highly substituted, insoluble protein fraction (7 and 47 hapten molecules per molecule of protein, respectively). The lightly substituted protein fraction appeared to produce better antisera. It is uncertain whether the effects observed related to the level of hapten substitution or to conjugate solubility. Despite this report, until further studies are carried out with haptens having varying degrees of structural complexity, it cannot be concluded that proteins that are lightly substituted with hapten are always or even usually preferable to heavily substituted proteins in immunoassay development. In the meantime, it seems desirable to continue to immunize with relatively heavily substituted conjugates (in the range of 5 to 15 haptenic groups per molecule of protein).

The Choice of a Protein for Conjugation

The choice of the protein for conjugation is influenced by commercial availability, immunogenicity, molecular size, solubility, and availability of functional groups. In our own studies we have always assumed that any protein would do, provided that it was immunogenic and that adequate conjugation could be achieved. Since protein amino groups are largely derived from ϵ-ammonium groups of lysine and protein carboxylate groups from the beta and gamma carboxyls of aspartic and glutamic acid, the number of potentially reactive groups for a given conjugation procedure is easily calculated from published molecular-weight and amino-acid-composition data for proteins. We have frequently used human or bovine serum albumin because both proteins have large numbers of amino groups and their solubility properties usually permit them to remain in solution under a variety of conditions of pH and ionic strength, in the presence of organic solvents and even after extensive cross linking. As noted, retention of full solubility after conjugation is not necessary for immunogenicity, but it does simplify the analysis if spectrophotometric methods are being used to determine the number of attached haptenic groups. We have also utilized keyhole limpet and limulus hemocyanin because of their unusual potency as immunogens. From a survey of the literature it is evident that a wide variety of other proteins, including bovine and chicken gamma globulin, bovine thyroblobulin, ovalbumin and bovine fibrinogen, are suitable as carriers for hapten. Skowsky and Fisher (quoted in Odell et al., 1971) have studied the immunogenicity of various protein and polyamino-acid conjugates of lysine vasopressin and triiodothyronine and advocate the use of bovine thyroglobulin as a carrier for hapten. Using the thyroglobulin conjugates, they obtained a good antibody response to the determinants in virtually all the animals tested, whereas no antibody response was obtained with bovine serum albumin, polylysine, and polyglutamic acid conjugates. Their observations are of considerable interest, for if bovine thyroglobulin is actually preferable to bovine serum albumin as a carrier, it should be used more extensively. Moreover, it might be desirable to make a systematic evaluation of other protein carriers, since thyroglobulin might not necessarily be optimal either. On the other hand, it is puzzling that Skowsky and Fisher failed to obtain antibodies to lysine vasopressin with BSA conjugates of the octapeptide, for in our own studies this combination not only produced antibodies but also permitted the development of a highly sensitive assay (Permutt et al., 1966). Based on this experience, it seems doubtful that there is as much difference between protein carriers as the work of Skowsky and Fisher would seem to suggest.

Nonprotein Carriers

There is ample evidence that the macromolecular carrier for the hapten need not necessarily be a protein in order to stimulate antibody formation. In fact, it has been argued that the use of synthetic polyaminoacids (Fig. 2.6) containing one or several selected amino acids and a sizable number of free carboxylate or amino groups may be advantageous in permitting a conjugation reaction that is more selective, gives a better-defined reaction product, minimizes possible antigenic competition, and eliminates possible confusion from antiprotein antibodies. Simple polyamino acids have been employed successfully as carriers in preparing antibodies to angiotensin,

$$
\begin{array}{ccc}
X \ \ O & Y \ \ O & Z \ \ O \\
| \ \ \| & | \ \ \| & | \ \ \| \\
..NH-CH-C-NH-CH-C-NH-CH-C... \\
R_1 & R_2 & R_3
\end{array}
$$

Fig. 2.6. General formula for a polyamino acid. X, Y, or Z may contain functional groups suitable for conjugation to a hapten.

prostaglandins, and luteinizing hormone-releasing factor (Haber, 1969; Levine et al., 1971; Hichens et al., 1974). Unfortunately, polyamino acid carriers sometimes fail to induce antihapten-antibody formation (Parker et al., 1962; Parker et al., 1965). In one study, repeated and prolonged attempts at immunization with tetrapeptide fragments of gastrin attached to positively or negatively charged polyamino acids were completely unsuccessful, whereas the same peptides attached to a foreign protein were highly immunogenic (Jaffe et al., 1970). Similar problems with polypeptide carriers have been encountered in attempting to immunize with bradykinin, triiodothyronine, and lysine vasopressin (Odell et al., 1971; Parker, 1971), and it is possible that numerous additional examples have not been reported. The negative examples are not surprising; as already indicated, the immunogenicity of the macromolecular carrier is critical in determining whether antihapten-antibodies are formed, and homo- or even heteropolymers of polyamino acids tend to be relatively poor immunogens. The advantage of avoiding the formation of antiprotein antibodies is highly problematical in any case, since all antisera contain hundreds or thousands of adventitious antibodies. Indeed, antibodies to the protein carrier do not complicate the assay, provided that the radioindicator molecule is not contaminated by carrier. Thus the advantages of using polyamino acid carriers are more apparent than real; and because of the uncertainty that they will promote immunization, normally they should not be used. One exception is the situation already discussed, where the goal is to conjugate a peptide to a carrier exclusively through its C-terminal end. With an ordinary protein, a carboxylate activating reagent would activate COOH groups on the protein as well as the peptide, and some of the peptide molecules would be attached through their amino terminal ends. In this case, the utilization of a polyamino acid containing lysyl but not glutamyl nor aspartyl residues in conjunction with a water-soluble carbodiimide will permit the desired conjugation reaction with little or no risk of conjugation through the opposite end of the peptide. There is little or no advantage in reversing the procedure (e.g., utilizing polymers containing glutamyl or aspartyl residues when conjugation through the amino terminal end of the polypeptide is desired) because of the availability of specific or highly selective coupling agents for amino groups (the bifunctional imidoesters and isocyanates) that permit a directed conjugation reaction with ordinary proteins.

The Introduction of Functional Groups onto Haptens
for Conjugation

Drugs already containing suitable functional residues, such as carboxylate (prostaglandins, barbiturates, and lysergic acid) or amino (amphetamines) groups, can be coupled directly to proteins. This approach is especially useful when the functional group being utilized for attachment is well removed from the area needed for immunological recognition. Where the hapten does not contain appropriate functional groups, or where those groups must be left undisturbed if maximal antibody specificity is to be obtained (see below), it may be necessary to add new functional groups to the hapten by organic synthesis. In the case of digitoxigenin, cyclic AMP, cyclic GMP, morphine, estrogen, testosterone, and aldosterone, this process has been accomplished by adding a free carboxyl group (Steiner et al., 1969; Steiner et al., 1972; Spector and Parker, 1970; Abraham and Grover, 1971). The location of the new group must be carefully considered, for it may greatly influence antibody affinity, specificity, and cross-reactivity. In forming antibodies to cAMP, for example, there was the problem of measuring cAMP in the presence of low levels of cGMP and much higher levels of ATP, ADP, and 5'-AMP. To maximize specificity,

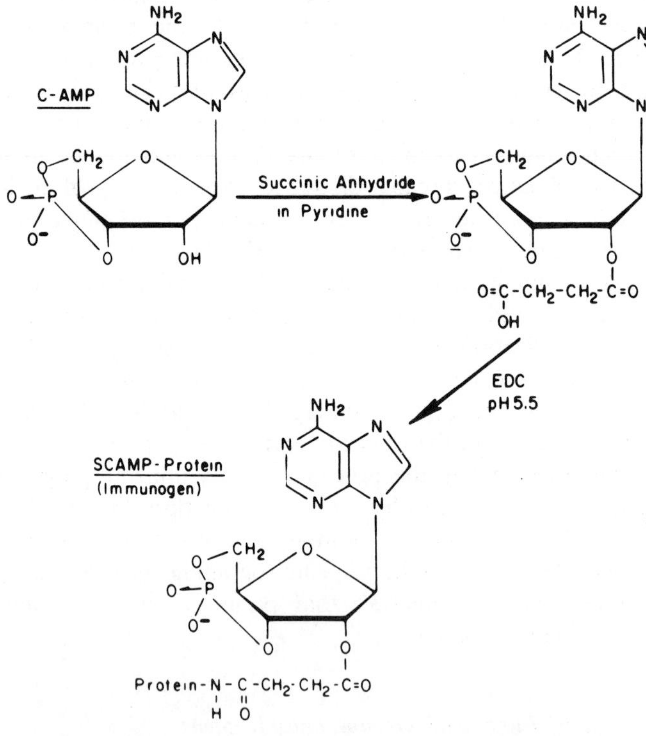

Fig. 2.7. Synthesis of 2'0-succinyl cyclic nucleotide and of cyclic nucleotide immunogen. SCAMP, succinylated cyclic AMP; EDC, 1-ethyl-3-(3-dimethyl-aminopropyl)-carbodiimide. (Taken from A. L. Steiner, C. W. Parker, and D. M. Kipnis. 1970. *In* P. Greengard, and E. Costa (Eds.). Advances in biochemical psychopharmacology. Vol. 3. Raven Press, New York. pp. 89–111.)

it seemed desirable to attach the cAMP to protein through the 2′O-position, leaving the phosphodiester group and the adenine ring unsubstituted and thus capable of contributing maximally to immunological specificity (Fig. 2.7). This was accomplished by succinylating cAMP at the 2′O-position and using the free carboxylate group of the succinate to attach the hapten to the protein carrier (Steiner et al., 1969; Parker, 1971). The specificity of an antibody obtained in this manner is shown in Fig. 2.8. When the

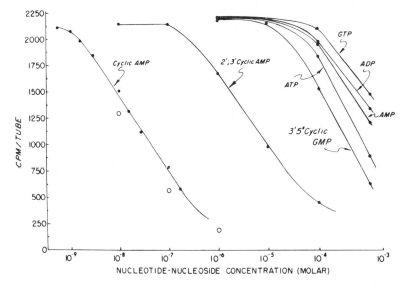

Fig. 2.8. The inhibition of ^{125}I-SCAMP-TME binding to cyclic AMP antibody by various nucleotides. o is 2′-deoxy 3′5′-cyclic AMP. (Taken from A. L. Steiner, D. M. Kipnis, R. Utiger, and C. Parker. 1969. Proc. Nat. Acad. Sci. USA. 64:373.)

quantities of nucleotide needed to inhibit the binding of the iodinated cyclic AMP marker were compared, cAMP produced a 50% reduction of binding at 10,000 to 1,000,000-fold lower concentrations than the other cyclic and noncyclic nucleotides. The only exception was 2′-3′-cyclic AMP, which inhibited binding at one hundredfold higher concentrations than cAMP (cross-reactivity of 0.01). Because of this low cross-reactivity, the direct immunoassay of cyclic AMP in tissue was possible without preliminary purification of the sample. Whether cAMP coupled to protein through one of the carbons or nitrogens in the purine ring system would have provided equally satisfactory antibodies seems highly unlikely, although this point has not been directly evaluated.

Another molecule that has a number of possible sites for the introduction of new functional groups or direct conjugation is morphine. Starting with the intact morphine, molecule attachment of the drug to protein is

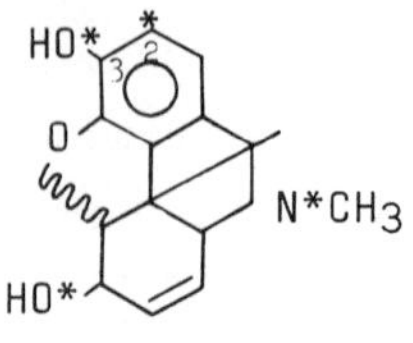

Morphine

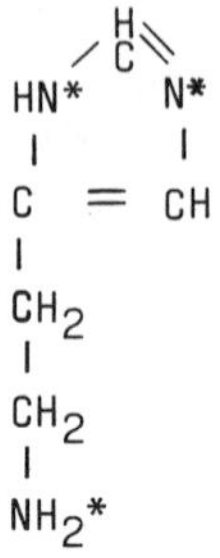

Histamine

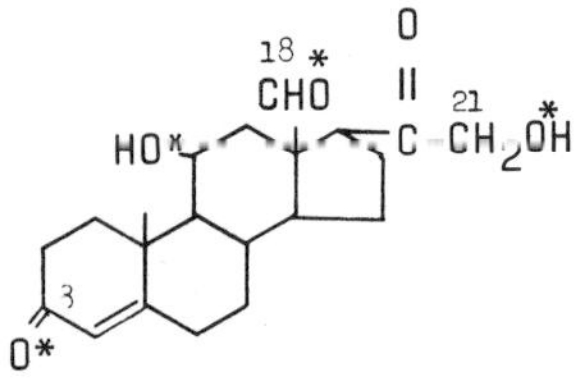

Aldosterone

Fig. 2.9. Structural formulas for morphine, histamine, and aldosterone. Sites readily available for conjugation are indicated by an asterisk.

possible through the phenolic hydroxyl group at position 3, the alcoholic hydroxyl group at position 6, and the N-methyl group or a diazo linkage at position 2 (Fig. 2.9). The method of conjugation chosen will influence the relative cross-reactivities of the various morphine congeners. For example, codeine, which is the 3-methyl ether of morphine, may react even better than morphine itself with antibodies to 3-carboxymethyl morphine (the latter also has a methylene group at the 3 position) (Spector and Parker, 1970). When morphine-6-hemisuccinate is used for immunization, morphine may be bound better than codeine, since the methyl group of codeine is not present on the immunogen (Wainer et al., 1973). Simultaneous immunoassays with the two types of antibodies provide a possible approach to the differentiation of morphine from codeine in an unknown sample, but with the antisera studied to date, the differences in codeine and morphine inhibition are sufficiently small that some form of preliminary separation is needed (Marks et al., 1974). Greater differences are seen in the binding of morphine-3-monoglucuronide, a metabolite of morphine. The glucuronide binds much better to antibodies to morphine-6-hemisuccinate than antibodies to 3-carboxymethyl morphine, presumably because of the greater steric hindrance to binding with the latter antibody (see below) (Spector et al., 1973).

Still another molecule that presents a choice of functional groups for conjugation is aldosterone, which can be linked to protein through a functional group added at C-3 through the keto residue or at C-21 through the OH residue (Fig. 2.9). In this case, with the expectation of conducting measurements of aldosterone in serum, conjugation through C-3 is clearly preferable, for it maximizes the specificity of the antibody for the opposite end of the molecule, which is where aldosterone differs structurally from other corticoids that circulate in the blood (Parker, 1971). For example, aldosterone differs from corticosterone only in having an aldehyde rather than a methyl group at position 18 (Fig. 2.9).

A final example is the problem presented in preparing antibodies to penicillin, as in developing an immunochemical procedure for measuring penicillin in body fluids. Here the question of potential immunological cross-reactivity is overriding. Penicillin can be coupled to protein amino groups through the carboxyl in the original four-membered B lactam ring of penicillin, thus resulting in the formation of a penicilloyl residue, which is an important antigenic determinant in human penicillin allergy (Parker, 1965a; Levine, 1965). It can also be coupled to protein through the carboxylate group on the sulfur-containing ring, leaving the lactam ring unaltered. Theoretically, the carboxylate conjugation is strongly preferred. Antibodies to penicilloyl recognize penicilloic acid, a hydrolysis product that accumulates in aqueous solutions of penicillin, much more readily than pencillin itself (a one hundredfold difference in immunological reactivity) (Thiel et al., 1964) and would have even greater reactivity for any protein-bound pencilloyl that might have formed. This problem can be avoided by use of the other method of conjugation.

When the haptenic group is small, finding a satisfactory mode of attachment to protein may offer serious difficulties. This problem arises both with epinephrine and histamine, and despite considerable effort, practical immunoassays are not yet available for either substance. Histamine, for example, is readily attached to protein either through its aliphatic amino groups via a conventional peptide bond or through one of the nitrogens on its imidazole ring via an azo linkage (Fig. 2.9). But both modes of attachment markedly alter one of the functional groups of histamine and diminish the potential specificity of any antibodies that might be obtained for unaltered histamine. Possible alternatives include attachment through a carbon on the imidazole ring of histamine, attachment through the carboxylate group of histidine, and attachment through the amino nitrogen of histamine by glutaraldehyde, followed by the reduction or the addition of a new functional group on the aliphatic side chain of histidine. The glutaraldehyde reduction procedure creates a secondary amino group at the position of the original histamine aliphatic amino group and restores the original positive charge. None of these approaches has been successful thus far, and it is possible that even with the best possible conjugation procedure imaginable, any antibodies obtained will have such low affinity for unaltered histamine that the development of a sensitive assay will not be possible.

In order to avoid deliberately synthesizing hapten derivatives with suitable functional groups for conjugation to protein, two other approaches are possible. In the past several months we have begun to explore the possible use of arylnitrenes to attach haptens or polypeptides to proteins. After exposure to light, nitrenes become extremely reactive chemically, acquiring the capability to insert into carbon hydrogen bonds and other locations that are normally very nonreactive (Knowles, 1972). Thus by the photocatalytic reaction of a nitrene with a hapten, substitutions can occur in areas of the hapten molecule that are not reactive to the usual coupling agents. If the nitrene is bifunctional, it can attach the hapten directly to the protein in a single-step procedure. If it contains a second functional residue, such as a carboxyl group, a two-step procedure can be used, reacting the hapten with the nitrene in the first step and employing one of the usual carboxylate activating agents with protein in the second step (Fig. 2.10). Haptens coupled in this way are certain to be heterogeneous, which is not necessarily a disadvantage, since the animal has a choice of coupled haptenic groups to which to mount an immune response. Alternatively, in the two-step reaction the initial hapten-nitrene reaction mixture can be fractionated before conjugation to protein and each of the products

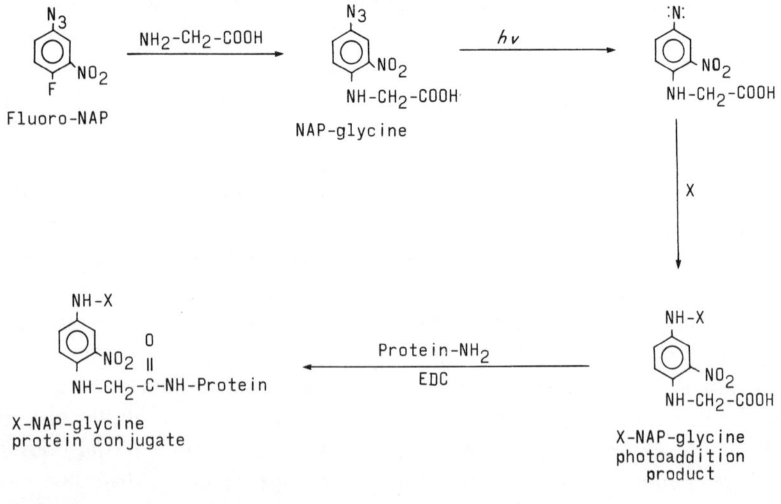

Fig. 2.10. Conjugation of a hapten to protein utilizing a photoactivatable nitrene group. The hapten is designated as X.

tested separately as an immunogen. A basically similar approach might involve exposing the hapten to a heavy pulse of ionizing radiation, thus creating free radical derivatives of the hapten. Free radicals have the capability of combining with protein, particularly at phenolic and sulfhydryl groups. As in the nitrene procedure, a heterogeneous product would almost certainly be obtained.

From the various examples given in this section it is apparent that the selection of a suitable conjugation procedure can be crucial in determining whether the needed sensitivity or specificity is achieved. Thus, depending on the purpose of the immunoassay and possible problems of cross-reactivity, one method of conjugation may be greatly preferable to another even though the two methods produce comparable quantities of antibody. When there is serious doubt as to the optimal method of conjugation or when antisera of differing specificities are needed, multiple methods of conjugation should be tried and optimal antisera identified empirically.

SUMMARY

1. Antibodies can be prepared to a seemingly endless number of substances, including proteins, polypeptides, carbohydrates, lipids, nucleic acids, heavy metals, drugs, and organic molecules of no known therapeutic value.

2. Small molecular weight substances (haptens) have little or no immunogenicity unless they are conjugated to an immunogenic carrier, usually a protein. Polyamino acids are less desirable as carriers because of the reduced likelihood that a useful antibody response will be obtained.

3. A wide variety of reagents are available for conjugating nonhaptenic molecules to proteins, the choice depending on the functional groups available on the hapten and the type of conjugation desired. Conjugation through the region of the molecule that is least important for immunologic recognition is important if antisera of maximal selectivity are to be obtained.

4. In attaching labile haptens to proteins, it is important to consider possible degradation of the hapten during conjugation, and this feature may influence the choice of the coupling reagent.

5. If the hapten does not contain a functional group suitable for conjugation to carrier, it can be introduced by organic synthesis.

6. In preparing hapten-protein conjugates for immunization, the goal is to introduce multiple haptenic groups on the protein. The exact level of substitution does not appear to be critical.

7. Antibody formation is possible to the coupling agent or protein carrier as well as to the hapten, and this situation is a possible source of misinterpretation.

Chapter 3

Immunization Procedures

Choosing an Animal Species

High-affinity antihapten antibodies ($K_a > 10^8$ liters/mole^{-1}, see below) can be obtained from rabbits, guinea pigs, goats, mice, and sheep, and it seems likely that the same capability exists in other species (Eisen, 1966; Odell et al., 1971). Systematic comparisons of antibody responses to the same antigen in different species have been limited. Moreover, it can be assumed that even where differences appear to exist, they may not hold for other antigens. Although large animals, such as goats, sheep, and horses, are effective antibody producers and provide large volumes of sera, most immunoassays can be performed with extremely small amounts of antibody. Therefore, in obtaining antisera, investigators have often chosen to work with the smaller, more easily handled laboratory animals, such as guinea pigs or rabbits. On rare occasions, one mammalian species appears to be greatly preferable to another in raising antisera, as seems to be true in the production of antisera to bovine insulin, where guinea pigs are the species of choice (Yalow and Berson, 1971). In immunizing with proteins with extensive areas of homology in different mammalian species, occasionally it is advantageous to immunize birds as well as mammals, in order to obtain as much of a phylogenic gap as possible (see below).

By and large, animals producing antibodies to endogenous hormones do not exhibit signs of hormonal insufficiency, probably because there is enough dissocation of the complexes to permit a continuing supply of hormone to the tissues. Under appropriate circumstances, however, antibody-mediated resistance to the in vivo action of insulin (Yalow and Berson, 1971), growth hormone (Parker and Daughaday, 1964), ACTH, TSH, HCG, or glucagon (Grey et al., 1970) can be demonstrated. Similar observations have been made with such drugs as morphine (Spector et al., 1973) and digitalis (Schmidt et al., 1974). Whether circulating hormones tie up the most avid antibodies, reducing the potential sensitivity of an antiserum for assay, is not known at present but is possible theoretically, particularly with hormones that circulate at relatively high concentrations.

24

THE PURITY OF THE IMMUNOGEN

Although the antigen should be as pure as possible, it need not necessarily be completely homogeneous. Even though antibody is formed to contaminants, if the antigen marker in the radioimmunoassay is highly purified and does not cross-react with the other proteins, there will be no interference in the assay. With proteins available in limited quantities, it is a much simpler matter to obtain the very small quantities needed for radiolabeling in a pure state than the larger quantities needed for immunization. The ability of the immune system to respond to multiple antigens simultaneously is evident from the multiplicity of antibodies that can be obtained in response to complex antigenic mixtures, such as serum. Some of the rabbit or goat antisera used for immunoelectrophoretic studies of human serum recognize as many as 25 to 30 distinct proteins. Indeed, Yalow and Berson (1971) have obtained useful antisera after immunization with crude gastrin preparations containing only 0.5% of the hormone. However, in other situations in which the immunogen is 10% or less of the total protein in the mixture, antigenic competition can occur, thereby leading to an unsatisfactory immune response. This situation is particularly likely to occur if the immunizing antigen is a poor immunogen and other stronger immunogens are present. In other words, relative immunogenicity among competing antigens is as important as their total number and individual concentrations (Parker, 1971). In dealing with a weak immunogen, extensive purification of the antigen may be required before a useful antiserum is obtained. Even a partial additional purification may be useful, since relative antigenic concentration is important in the degree of competition obtained.

Although the mechanism of antigenic competition is not entirely clear, it is of interest that when antibody synthesis is markedly depressed, there can be adverse effects on antibody affinities as well as concentrations. Harel et al. (1970) observed a moderate but significant depression of the average affinity of anti-DNP antibodies obtained from guinea pigs immunized with a mixture of DNP-bovine serum albumin and bovine gamma globulin in complete Freund's adjuvant. Kim et al. (1974) obtained similar results when antibody synthesis was depressed to a comparable degree (90% or more) but observed little or no effect when antibody synthesis was depressed only 30% (Werblin and Siskind, 1972). Whether animals with depressed antibody affinities eventually form maximal affinity antibodies if the immunization is sustained long enough is not yet known.

Contaminants that cross-react immunologically with the immunogen sometimes pose more of a problem than non-cross-reacting contaminants. Antisera may recognize the contaminant as well or better than the principal immunogen, and attempts to improve antiserum specificity by absorption with the cross-reacting protein or hapten may remove a portion of the antibody to the homologous antigen. The purity of the immunogen is especially important with synthetic peptides because of possible contamination with "error peptides," which are partially racemized or contain incorrect amino acid sequences or incompletely removed blocking groups (Playfair et al., 1974). Despite the desirability of eliminating cross-reacting antigens, useful antiprotein- or antipolypeptide-antigen antisera can sometimes be obtained by immunization with crude tissue extracts containing several cross-reacting proteins. For example, antibodies to porcine β-MSH have been prepared for immunoassay use by immunization with commercial porcine ACTH, which is heavy contaminated with β-MSH (Orth, 1974). Useful antisera are also obtained with partially purified FSH and LH, cross-reacting hormones that almost invariably contaminate one another (Odell et al., 1971). Success with this approach requires that the antisera be absorbed with the cross-reacting hormone and that large num bers of sera be screened.

THE PURPOSE OF THE IMMUNOLOGICAL ADJUVANT

Just prior to immunization, the antigen is usually incorporated in a water-in-oil emulsion containing either human or bovine Mycobacteria, (complete Freund's adjuvant). (The preparation of the emulsion is described in Williams and Chase, 1967.) The use of the water-in-oil emulsion helps stimulate immune reactivity. It also partially protects labile antigens—favoring immunization with readily degradable substances having a very short half life in serum—and delays the absorption of the antigen, thus permitting a reduction in frequency of booster injections (Parker, 1971). Mycobacteria increase the inflammatory response in regional nodes, amplifying the immune response and helping stimulate the eventual formation of high-affinity antibody. Microorganisms other than Mycobacteria also potentiate immune responsiveness and may be considered if the results with Mycobacteria are disappointing. However, evidence for selectivity in adjuvant action is inconclusive and probably not sufficient to justify trials with several different bacterial or chemical adjuvants each time a new immunogen is evaluated.

IMMUNOGEN ADMINISTRATION AND DOSAGE

Immunization with small-to-moderate amounts of antigen in complete adjuvant favors the development of a sustained immune response and the eventual elaboration of an antibody with a high affinity for the antigen.

This situation is especially well documented for immune responses to haptens (Eisen and Siskind, 1964; Werblin and Siskind, 1972) but appears to apply to a variety of other immunogens, including proteins (Urbain et al., 1972) and polysaccharides (Kimball, 1972). For most species and antigens, the optimal quantity of antigen for a full course of immunization is in the range of 0.1 to 1.0 mg/kg body weight. The amount of antigen administered may need to be adjusted upward if an impure antigen mixture or an unconjugated small molecular weight polypeptide is being given. When the amount of antigen available for immunization is very limited, much smaller doses can sometimes be used with good results, particularly if the antigen is relatively pure. Thus antibodies to carcinoembryonic antigen suitable for immunoassay use were obtained after immunization of goats with a total dose of 31 μg of antigen per animal (Egan et al., 1972). Relatively young but essentially full-grown animals are preferred. The immunization is best given in the form of multiple (6 to 8), small (0.05 to 0.10 ml), intradermal or subcutaneous injections, usually including the toe-pads (wherever feasible). About 50% of the total antigen dose is given at the time of the primary injection. When toe pad injections are given, local inflammation may be a problem but can be reduced by the use of relatively small injection volumes and a diminution in the quantity of Mycobacteria in the adjuvant. When unusually small quantities of immunogen are available, the method of Vaitukaitis et al. (1971), in which immunogen is given intradermally in complete Freund's adjuvant in some 30 to 50 intradermal sites, may be advantageous. In addition to stimulating a substantial response with small quantities of immunogen, it has been suggested that the method provides for more rapid formation of antibody (Playfair et al., 1974). However, at conventional doses of immunogen, Marks et al. (1974) failed to obtain a quicker or more avid antibody response via this method.

Booster injections, smaller in quantity (approximately 5 to 10% of the initial dose) but identical in composition (adjuvant, protein carrier,* coupling agent, level of hapten substitution), are administered intermit-

---

* The generalization that the same protein carrier and coupling agent should be used throughout the immunization may eventually have to be modified. It is now clear that late in the course of immunization (after 4 to 6 months), haptens attached to heterologous protein carriers may stimulate booster responses and that the antibody obtained has a high affinity for the hapten (Werblin and Siskind, 1972). On the other hand, by reinjection of the original hapten-protein conjugate, high-affinity antihapten antibody also is obtained and the overall response is greater. Which procedure is better for maximizing affinity is not yet clear, but in view of extensive and generally favorable experience with repeated injections of primary conjugates, they should continue to be used until a definitive comparison is made.

tently over a period of months (Parker, 1971). Injections for boosting should be given at sites that restimulate lymph nodes that are involved in the primary response. Therefore areas near the original injection sites should be used for secondary stimulation unless exceptionally marked local inflammation precludes their use. During immunization with proteins or hapten-protein conjugates, booster injections are given about every 6 weeks. More frequent injections are not necessary, for during the first 4 to 6 weeks of immunization it is difficult to demonstrate further increases in antibody titer after boosting. Presumably the immunological apparatus is already being stimulated optimally by residual antigen from the primary injection, and it is only after the level of antigen has fallen further that clear-cut booster effects are obtained. In the case of unconjugated polypeptides, readministration of the immunogen every 1 to 2 weeks is desirable to replace immunogen that has been excreted or degraded. In preparation for boosting with hapten-protein conjugates, it is important to consider possible deterioration of the conjugate during storage, and it may be desirable to prepare a fresh conjugate.

DURATION OF IMMUNIZATION

Immunized animals are bled serially, usually 4 to 10 days after each booster injection, beginning at about 6 to 8 weeks after immunization. Since the use of complete adjuvant favors a sustained response, the time of harvesting normally is not critical. Rabbits can be bled from the ears with very little risk of losing the animal. As a rule, the best antisera are obtained after immunization has been in progress for 3 to 8 months. However, in the absence of previous experience with an immunogen, it is not always possible to predict when high-affinity, high-titer antibody will be present. Enough variation in the immune response from animal to animal exists to make it desirable that each serum sample be examined separately. This step is particularly important when antigenic cross-reactivity is a potential problem. In general, animals that produce good antisera (in terms of titer and specificity) early in the immune response provide the best antisera in later bleedings, and generally it is not desirable to continue to immunize poorly responding animals. The specificity of late antibodies can differ from that of earlier antibodies from the same animal; and even if a late antiserum appears satisfactory for immunoassay use on other grounds, it will be necessary to reverify the specificity. Late in the course of immunization there may be a fall in average antibody affinity, but after restimulation with antigen, a rapid and selective increase in the concentration of high-affinity antibodies usually occurs (Werblin and Siskind, 1972; Urbain et al., 1972). Interestingly, if animals immunized initially with high doses of antigen are followed long enough, they eventually make high-affinity antibodies (Kim and Siskind, 1974). Thus low doses of antigen favor early selection for high-affinity antibody synthesis, whereas large doses of antigen lead to slower selection, extending over a period of many months.

A considerable variation in the rate of maturation of the immune response is evident when responses to proteins or polypeptides are compared with those to haptens. Sera that are satisfactory for the immunoassay of human protein-polypeptide hormones have been obtained after only 4 to 6 weeks of immunization of guinea pigs in complete adjuvant, although later antisera are often even better. A representative immune response with human FSH is shown in Fig. 3.1. An immunization-dose respond curve for the same immunogen is given in Fig. 3.2. Additional

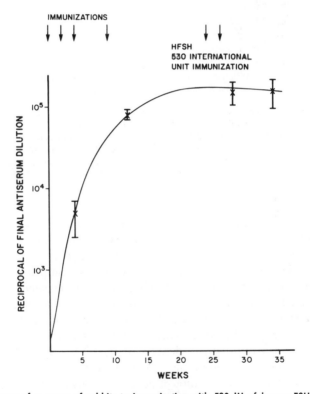

Fig. 3.1. Response of a group of rabbits to immunization with 530 IU of human FSH. Note that the titer plateaus at just over 1:100,000. The quantity of protein in milligrams was not specified, but human FSH contains maximally about 2,000 units/mg protein. (Taken from W. D. Odell, G. A. Abraham, W. R. Skowsky, M. A. Hescox, and D. A. Fisher. 1971. *In* W. D. Odell, and W. H. Daughaday (Eds.). Principles of competitive protein-binding assays. J. B. Lippincott Co., Philadelphia. pp. 57–76.)

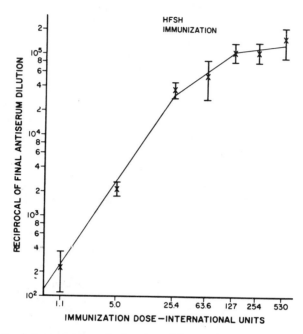

Fig. 3.2. Relation between the immunization dose of human FSH administered every 10 to 14 days in complete Freund's adjuvant and the titer obtained after five injections. Note that with doses greater than 127 IU, the titer did not increase further. For discussion of quantity of protein in milligrams, see Fig. 3.1. (Taken from W. D. Odell, G. A. Abraham, W. R. Skowsky, M. A. Hescox, and D. A. Fisher. 1971. *In* W. D. Odell, and W. H. Daughaday (Eds.). Principles of competitive protein-binding assays. J. B. Lippincott Co., Philadelphia. pp. 57–76.)

data on responses to polypeptide or protein hormones appear in Table 3.1. Antihapten sera are usually not optimal for immunoassay application until 4 to 6 months have elapsed. With large hydrophobic haptens, the delay may be even longer. For example, useful antiprostaglandin antibodies were not obtained until after one year of repeated immunization (Jaffe et al., 1971; Jaffe et al., 1973). Marked delays in maturation of the immune response have also been observed in the production of antibodies to such steroids as digitoxin (Oliver et al., 1968), aldosterone (Oliver et al., 1971), estrogen, and 11-desoxycortisol (Odell et al., 1971). Representative curves for estradiol and 11-desoxycortisol are given in Fig. 3.3 (compare with Fig. 3.1). Although generalizations are difficult, if antisera that meet the sensitivity requirements of the immunoassay are not obtained within 6 to 12 weeks, it may be worthwhile to continue the immunization, particularly if a structurally complex hapten is involved.

The time required to generate a useful antiserum is not solely dependent on the pattern of the immune response. As discussed below, the assay requirements in terms of maximization of affinity may be considerably higher for haptens than for proteins, thereby increasing the necessity for utilizing optimal immunization procedures. This is based in part on the fact that proteins undergo multivalent interactions with antibody, whereas haptens react univalently.

Table 3.1

Representative, currently recommended immunization procedures for obtaining useful antisera to unconjugated human or animal polypeptide hormones.

Immunogen	Animal	Minimal initial dose (mg protein)	Minimal total dose (mg protein)	Number injections	Time of high titer (weeks)	Representative titer (50% precipitation Ag)
H-GH	GP	0.5	3.5	5	12-16	1:50,000
H-TSG	R	0.1	0.3	2-3	3-4	1:100,000
P-In	GP	5.0	10.0	2-3	6-9	1:32,000
O-PRL	GP	0.5	0.6	2-6	4-8	1:40,000
H-LH	R	1.0	5.0	4	7-10	1:15,000
H-CG	R	0.2 *	0.6 *	3	6	1:500,000
H-PL	GP, R	1.0	1.5	3	8	1:200,000

Taken from the appropriate sections in Jaffe and Berman (1974).

Abbreviations H-GH (human growth hormone); H-TSH (human thyrotrophic hormone); P-In (Porcine insulin); O-PRL (ovine prolactin); H-LH (human luteinizing hormone); H-CG (human chorionic gonadotrophin); H-PL (human placental lactogen); R (rabbit); GP (guinea pig).

* Estimated from the stated quantity of hormone units assuming 15,000 IU/mg.

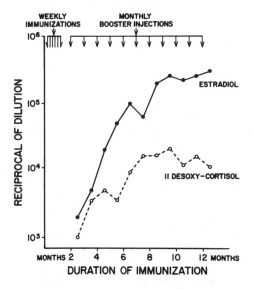

Fig. 3.3. Response of two sheep immunized with steroid-albumin conjugates. Note that titer plateaued at 8 to 9 months. (Taken from W. D. Odell, G. A. Abraham, W. R. Skowsky, M. A. Hescox, and D. A. Fisher. 1971. In W. D. Odell, and W. H. Daughaday (Eds.). Principles of competitive protein-binding assays. J. B. Lippincott Co., Philadelphia. pp. 57–76.)

THE THEORETICAL BASIS
FOR IMMUNOLOGICAL MATURATION

The influence of antigen dose and duration of immunization is most easily visualized as an effect of cell selection (Eisen and Siskind, 1964; Werblin and Siskind, 1972). It is assumed that every animal contains many different subpopulations of antigen-sensitive lymphocytes, each with the predetermined capability of responding to one or a limited number of antigens. The cells involved have surface receptors for antigen and are stimulated to replicate when an optimal number of antigen molecules becomes attached. The result is an intense proliferative response that greatly expands the population of antigen-sensitive cells. Many of the new cells that are generated are antibody-producing cells, and as the number of these cells increases, serum antibody becomes demonstrable. If all the antibody-producing cells gave rise to antibodies with identical binding properties, there would be no opportunity to modulate the immune response by altering the immunization conditions. However, even with apparently homogeneous antigens, the affinity of the antibody for antigen varies over a broad range. The binding heterogeneity is due to differences among the cells that make the antibody. It is assumed that cells synthesizing high-affinity antibodies have high-affinity receptors and are optimally stimulated at low concentrations of antigen, whereas the cells producing low-affinity antibodies are optimally stimulated at high antigen concentrations. Thus when low antigen doses are to be used, the formation of high-affinity antibodies is favored, whereas with high antigen doses much of the antibody is of the low-affinity variety. The effect of immunization duration relates to a need for continuing antigen stimulation throughout the immunization period. Antibody-producing cells replicate for a limited period and then die. Release of further antigen from the adjuvant continues the response, but since the concentration of antigen is gradually falling (in the absence of further boosting), eventually conditions of low antigen dose stimulation will prevail, thus maximizing the amount of high-affinity antibody formed. Studies with lymph node lymphocytes in tissue culture provide direct evidence that as the time after immunization increases, antibodies of increasing affinity are secreted (Steiner and Eisen, 1967). Another effect of prolonging the immunization is to provide ample time for the maximum expansion of the cells producing high-affinity antibody.

In the production of antihapten antibodies, the protein or polyamino acid carrier influences the magnitude and mode of evolution of the response. The reason that a macromolecule-bound hapten is immunogenic, whereas an unconjugated hapten is not, has not been completely clarified. Conjugation to protein delays the excretion of the hapten, but it is almost certainly not the mechanism. The immunogenicity of the protein component of the conjugate is important, since haptens that are attached to foreign proteins are more effective immunogens than haptens on native proteins. An attractive possibility is that the immunological activation is a sequential process in which the initial response is to the protein moiety. According to this view, hapten-protein conjugates act initially on thymus-dependent (T) lymphocytes with recognition sites for the protein. T lymphocytes that bind to the hapten-protein conjugate are stimulated and somehow recruit cells that are capable of forming antihapten antibody (B cells) (Mitchison, 1967; Katz and Benacerraf, 1972). In addition to the important role of T cells in promoting B cell activation, some polymeric antigens, such as polysaccharides, appear to be able to stimulate B cells directly. A protein carrier is required in the production of an anamestic response as well as in the primary immunization; and in order to obtain a maximal booster effect, the protein involved in the original immunization must be used. However, late in the response, some cells develop a high enough affinity for the hapten that triggering can take place with hapten-heterologous carrier conjugates, the magnitude of the response depending in part on the multiplicity of hapten groups per molecule of carrier. Thus there is a partial loss of carrier dependency late in the course of immunization.

Cell selection from a diverse population of preexisting antigen-sensitive cells is not the only mechanism that would explain the variation in the antibody response with time after immunization. Conceivably, the antigen-sensitive cells themselves undergo modulation in response to selective antigen pressures, producing better and better products by successive approximation until some practical limit is reached. This process might occur through an exchange of genetic information between cells or an unexplained ability on the part of responding antigen-sensitive cells to generate new cell lines with differing antigen-binding capabilities. This possibility receives some support from studies in tadpoles, where the number of available lymphocytes is very limited ($\sim 2 \times 10^6$) but the capacity to respond to many different antigens still exists. A simple cell selection theory also has difficulty in explaining why substantial amounts of low-affinity antibodies continue to be formed even very late in the immune response (Werblin and Siskind, 1972) and why very low antigen doses do not necessarily stimulate higher-affinity antibodies than intermediate doses that stimulate a maximal antibody response (Segre and Segre, 1973). Moreover, Marcario et al. (1972) have observed that small lymph node fragments from primed rabbits, believed to contain one or several clones of memory cells, elaborate antibodies of increasing affinity during a 40-day period of cultivation in vitro. Thus some factor in addition to clonal selection may be needed to explain the way in which the immune response evolves.

Regardless of the mechanism of immunologic maturation, it would appear that there is a ceiling on antibody affinity in a given animal. Under optimal conditions of immunization the level reached will ultimately depend on the genetic capacity of the animal to respond. After immunization for 6 months to a year, there may even be a fall in antibody titer or affinity, (C. W. Parker, unpublished observations; Kimball, 1972). The inability of some animals to sustain an optimal immune response indefinitely creates a difficult decision as to whether to bleed out the animal or continue to immunize and obtain smaller amounts of blood in the hope that the binding properties of the antibody will continue to improve.

The basis for the limitation in antibody affinity is uncertain. Theoretically, it is possible that as antibodies with very high affinities are synthesized, they form essentially irreversible complexes with antigen and are eliminated. It seems much more likely that the restriction is at the level of the antibody-producing cells themselves and the type of antibodies they are capable of producing.

SUMMARY

1. Antisera that are suitable for immunoassay use can be obtained from a variety of animal species. Unless unusually large volumes of sera are needed, rabbits, guinea pigs, or goats are normally the animals of choice. The use of relatively small animals is advantageous if only small quantities of immunogen are available, since the total dose for immunization is predicated on the size of the animal.

2. The immunogen is administered in adjuvant at multiple injection sites. The adjuvant not only eliminates the need for frequent injections and favors the development of high-affinity antibodies but may also help protect labile immunogens from rapid degradation. When unusually small quantities of immunogen are available, the use of a large number (30 to 50) of intradermal injection sites on the back and thighs may help to magnify the response. Intermediate rather than high doses of immunogen favor the development of a high-affinity response.

3. Because of possible antigenic competition or interference by cross-reacting antibodies in the immunoassay, pure antigens should be used wherever possible for immunization. Nonetheless, useful antisera can frequently be obtained by immunization with impure antigens. Contaminating antibodies do not interfere in the radioimmunoassay unless the antigen marker is also contaminated or a portion of the antibodies is directed toward cross-reacting antigen.

4. After immunization with protein and polypeptide immunogens, antisera that are suitable for immunoassay use are generally obtained within the first several months. The generation of effective antihapten antisera

usually takes longer, rarely as long as 8 months to a year. Ultimately a ceiling on antibody affinity is reached, and further immunization may produce less desirable antisera. In general, animals that are the best antibody producers early in the response continue to be more effective as the immunization is prolonged.

Chapter 4

Immunologic Specificity and Cross-Reactivity

HAPTENIC SPECIFICITY

Quantitative Methods for Expressing
the Antibody-Hapten Interaction

The reaction between antibody and antigen (or, more strictly, antibody and univalent hapten, since the mathematical treatment is simplified) is a simple, reversible reaction

$$(1) \qquad Ab + H \; \rightleftharpoons \; Ab \cdot H$$

where Ab, H, and Ab·H are the molar concentrations of free antibody sites, free hapten, and antibody-bound hapten, respectively. The stability of the complex at equilibrium is described mathematically by K_a, the association constant (given in liters mole^{-1}),

$$(2) \qquad K_a \; = \; \frac{(Ab \cdot H)}{(Ab)(H)}$$

Equation (2) for the reversible interaction between hapten and antibody may be also written as

$$(3) \qquad \Delta F^\circ = -RT \quad L_n K_a$$

where ΔF° is the standard free energy of the antibody-hapten interaction, R is the gas constant, T is the absolute temperature, and $L_n K_a$ is the natural logarithm of the association constant (note that the same symbol, R, is used in a different context below). A high-affinity antibody forms a relatively stable complex with antibody, with limited dissociation of the bond under physiologic conditions. Quantitatively, this situation is reflected by a high value for K_a and a large negative value for ΔF°. The presentation of hapten binding in terms of K_a and ΔF° is useful in the present discussion in that it provides a quantitative index of absolute binding energy and cross-reactivity.

36

General Features of Antibody-Hapten Interactions

Beginning with the early studies of Obermayer and Pick (1904) and Landsteiner (summarized in 1936), a vast number of empirical studies that define various features of antibody-hapten reactions have been carried out. The overall conclusions that have been reached from these studies are summarized below.

IMMUNOLOGIC COMPLEMENTARITY AND CROSS-REACTIVITY

An antibody nearly always reacts more effectively with the immunizing (homologous) antigen than with structurally related antigens. Thus when Little and Eisen (1966, 1967) immunized rabbits with the 2,4-dinitrophenyl (DNP) group, they found that the antibodies had a higher affinity for DNP than for the 2,4,6-trinitrophenyl (TNP) ligands despite their close chemical similarity:

$$O_2N-C_6H_2(NO_2)(NO_2)-NH-(CH_2)_4-CH(COOH)(NH_2)$$

TNP

$$O_2N-C_6H_3(NO_2)-NH-(CH_2)_4-CH(COOH)(NH_2)$$

DNP

When TNP was the immunogen, the converse was true, with better binding for TNP than DNP (Table 4.1). Not only was the specificity of the antibody population as a whole greater for the homologous hapten, but when anti-TNP antibodies were purified by specific precipitation with a DNP protein and elution with dinitrophenol to select for a small fraction of the total anti-TNP antibody with maximal specificity for DNP, the binding also continued to favor TNP (even though the difference was less striking than in the original antibody population). When anti-DNP antibodies were purified to select for maximal TNP binding, once again the homologous hapten (in this case, DNP) was bound more effectively. The anti-

Table 4.1

Relative association constants for TNP-aminocaproate and DNP-aminocaproate with two preparations of purified anti-TNP antibody obtained at different times after immunization.

	5 weeks after immunization		10 weeks after immunization	
	K_0 (M^{-1})	$-\Delta F°$	K_0 (M^{-1})	$-\Delta F°$
TNP-aminocaproate	151×10^6	11.3	347×10^6	11.8
DNP-aminocaproate	0.9×10^6	8.3	26.3×10^6	10.3

K_0 and $-\Delta F°$ are the average association constants and standard free energies of binding, respectively, as determined by fluorescence quenching. (Taken from Little and Eisen, 1966.)

bodies also exhibited subtle structural differences in that the fluorescence of rabbit anti-TNP antibodies was less susceptible to quenching by either TNP or DNP ligands than the DNP antibodies. This finding was true even with antibodies selected for maximal DNP cross-reactivity as described above and after animals that had been immunized with TNP were boosted with DNP. Thus despite the marked structural similarity and immunologic cross-reactivity between TNP and DNP, the two haptens elicit antibodies that are easily distinguishable both structurally and functionally.

Immunological cross-reactivity similar to that displayed by TNP and DNP is seen with other antihapten antibodies, the relative reactivity of structural analogs of the hapten being dependent on their physicochemical properties and three-dimensional structure in so far as they approximate those of the immunizing hapten. Antibodies exhibit stereospecific binding and distinguish between the homologous optical enantiomorph and its stereoisomers. The importance of three-dimensional structure in binding has led to the general concept of structural complementarity between antibody and hapten.

INDIVIDUAL ANTISERUM VARIATION IN ANTIBODY
COMPLEMENTARITY AND CROSS-REACTIVITY

Antibodies from different animals vary markedly in their degree of cross-reactivity with structurally related haptens. In serial bleedings from the same animal, antisera that show minimal cross-reactivity early tend to have limited cross-reactivity at later times, although this is not always true. Antibodies of high affinity generally show greater cross-reactivity than antibodies of low affinity (Table 4.1, comparing the difference in $-\Delta F$s for TNP and DNP for the 5-week and 10-week antibodies). Since antibody affinity ordinarily rises with time after immunization, cross-reactivity also tends to increase and will be at or close to a maximum in the high-affinity antisera used in sensitive immunoassays. Fortunately, in competitive binding measurements, the increase in cross-reactivity with increasing antibody affinity is not as marked as would otherwise appear because the marker is also bound more effectively.

THE ROLE OF HAPTEN STRUCTURE IN ANTIBODY AFFINITY
AND CROSS-REACTIVITY

Antibodies to large, hydrophobic haptens tend to have a higher average affinity for the homologous hapten than antibodies to hydrophilic determinants (Table 4.2), probably because of the large change in free

Table 4.2

Range of association constants of antihapten antibodies.

Hapten	Apparent average K_a (liters/mole)
p-azophenyl lactoside	8×10^6
Pneumococcal polysaccharide, Type VIII	3×10^5
2,4-Dinitrophenyl-lysine	1×10^8
Dichlorofluorescein	1×10^{10}
Digitoxin, digoxin	1×10^{10}
Dansyl	1×10^8
NIP	3×10^7

Representative average association constants of different antihapten antibodies obtained from hyperimmunized rabbits or horses. Association constants were determined by equilibrium dialysis or fluorescence quenching. NIP is the 3-nitro-4-hydroxy-5-nitrophenyl acetyl group. Note the greater than 3 log variation in the association constant. Since identical immunization procedures were not used, the differences may partly reflect the mode of immunization, but this is almost certainly not the full explanation.

energy involved in transferring a nonpolar molecule from a hydrophobic environment into aqueous solution (Karush, 1962). They also exhibit greater immunologic cross-reactivity with structurally related haptens than antibodies to more polar determinants (more than would be predicted on the basis of absolute increases in antibody affinity per se). Indeed, low levels of binding affinity may be exhibited for hydrophobic molecules that are not structural analogs of the homologous hapten (Parker and Osterland, 1970). This finding is especially notable with certain mouse or human myeloma proteins that bind to DNP groups but also have considerable affinity for vitamin K and its congeners and 5-acetyl uracil; these latter structures are also hydrophobic but otherwise bear relatively little structural resemblance to DNP (Underdown and Eisen, 1971). Some of these proteins even bind effectively to DNA (Riesen and Castel, 1973). Because nonspecific binding can occur, antibodies to hydrophobic haptens need to be checked carefully for unexpected cross-reactivities, particularly since hydrophobic molecules, such as cholesterol, circulate in the blood at high concentrations. Nonetheless, as used operationally, even antibodies to hydrophobic haptens normally exhibit remarkable binding specificity, and structurally unrelated hydrophobic molecules rarely present problems.

ANTIBODY RESPONSES TO STRUCTURALLY COMPLEX HAPTENS

Antibodies to small haptenic groups show specificity for the amino acid side chain to which the hapten is attached on the immunizing protein as well as to the hapten itself (Eisen and Siskind, 1964). Thus antibodies to DNP-substituted proteins bind especially well to ε-DNP-lysine because, on DNP proteins, DNP substitution is primarily on lysyl residues of the protein (Eisen, 1966). And as shown in Fig. 4.1, in a homologous series

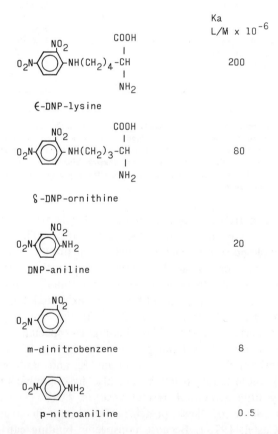

Fig. 4.1. Contribution of the amino acid side chain to the binding of ε-DNP-lysine by rabbit anti-DNP antibody. Based on data presented by Eisen and Siskind (1964).

of DNP derivatives, the closer the structural similarity to ϵ-DNP-lysine, the better the binding.

Antibodies to haptens that occupy a large volume generally have specificity for only a portion of the total molecule. When a chemically well-defined hapten-protein conjugate is used for immunization, the area of the hapten that is farthest away from the point of attachment to protein usually dominates the immunological specificity (e.g., contributes the most to overall binding energy) and can therefore be termed the immunodominant region. This is particularly true when the terminal residue itself is an effective immunogen, as illustrated (Fig. 4.2) by the *p*-azophenyl lactoside (Lac) group (Karush, 1957). *P*-nitrophenyl B-lactoside, which is structurally equivalent to the outer three-fourths of the immunizing hapten,

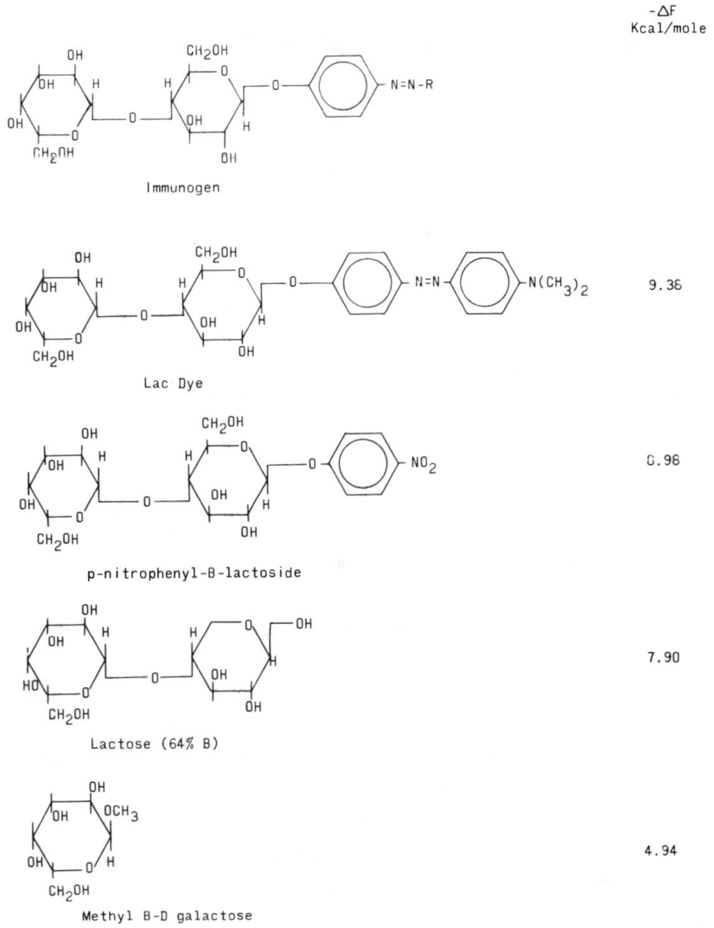

Fig. 4.2. Contributions of different portions of the Lac hapten to binding by rabbit anti-Lac antibody. Based on data presented by Karush (1957).

was bound nearly as well as the immunizing hapten, as shown by its high negative free energy of binding. With decreasing proportions of the original hapten available for binding (lactose and methyl-B-D-galactose), binding energy progressively decreased, although even methyl-B-D-galactose exhibited appreciable binding. Thus most of the antibodies have specificity for the two-terminal monosaccharide residues and the phenolic ring that connects them to the protein.

The general rule that terminal residues dominate the immune response has important exceptions, as exhibited by studies we conducted some years ago (Parker et al., 1966) with a DNP-tetrapeptide antigen, Val-ϵ-DNP-Lys-Leu-Phe-OEt (Table 4.3). The DNP peptide was coupled to protein

Table 4.3

Binding of various DNP derivatives by purified rabbit antibodies.

		K_0 (liters mole^{-1} $\times$ 10^{-6})		
No.	Hapten	LT-A	LT-B	Anti-DNP BγG
I	Val-ϵ-DNP-Lys-Leu-Phe-OEt	110.0	50.0	80.0
II	Val-ϵ-DNP-Lys-Gly-Phe-OEt	100.0	150.0	200.0
III	Val-ϵ-DNP-Lys-Gly-Gly-OEt	12.0	180.0	300.0
IV	Val-ϵ-DNP-Lys-OMe	10.0	230.0	300.0
V	ϵ-DNP-L-lysine	5.0	160.0	320.0
VI	γ-DNP-α-γ-diaminobutyrate	0.6	19.0	110.0
VII	ϵ-DNP-D-lysine	4.5	150.0	300.0

LT-A and LT-B were purified rabbit antibodies from individual animals immunized with HSA-Val-DNP-Lys-Leu-Phe-OEt (L-L-L-L, by absorption and elution from a DNP protein that did not contain the remainder of the peptide). The anti-DNP-BγG antibody was purified in the same way from a pool of rabbit antisera to DNP-BγG. All the antisera were obtained 8 to 9 weeks after immunization. Average association constants were determined by fluorescence quenching of purified anti-DNP antibodies. The fluorometric titrations were carried out in 0.15 M NaCl-0.01 M phosphate, pH 5.75, at 30°C. All amino acid residues were in the L-configuration unless otherwise specified. (Taken from Parker, Godt, and Johnson, 1966.)

through its N-terminal end, thus positioning the DNP group two amino acid residues away from the penultimate amino acid residue. Despite the internal location of the DNP group, anti-DNP antibodies were obtained that could be purified by precipitation with DNP proteins that did not contain the remainder of the peptide. The purified anti-DNP-tetrapeptide antibodies not only had a high affinity for ϵ-DNP-lysine, but they also sometimes displayed binding specificity for other regions of the peptide. Thus with one of the two anti-DNP-tetrapeptide antibodies shown in Table 4.3, the side chain of phenylalanine contributed up to 1.6 kcal of binding energy to overall tetrapeptide binding, (antibody LT-A, comparing the binding of the tetrapeptide with that of Val-DNP-Lys-Gly-Phe-OEt and Val-DNP-Lys-Gly-Gly-OEt). The phenylalanine side chain projects from the same side of the peptide as the DNP group, whereas the leucyl side chain, which is closer to the DNP group but does not contribute to binding, projects in the opposite direction. With the other antitetrapeptide antibody (LT-B), the presence of the phenylalanine side chain actually resulted in decreased ligand binding. One implication of these studies is that, with relatively small haptens, an immune response can occur to a combined determinant in which the hapten, the amino acid to which it is attached, and contiguous amino acids all contribute, but this situation is influenced to a great extent by the animal involved in the response (see below).

ANTIBODY HETEROGENEITY

Antibodies to haptens normally display marked binding heterogeneity, even when they are separated into individual immunoglobulin classes and are obtained as a single bleeding from an individual animal. With suitable fractionation techniques, antibody subpopulations that have differing affinities for homologous hapten and varying degrees of cross-reactivity for structurally related molecules can be obtained (Eisen and Siskind, 1964). In individual sera, the association constant of antibody for the homologous hapten may vary by as much as four orders of magnitude. The available data indicate that antibody heterogeneity is due in part to the use of non-homogeneous antigens for immunization and in part to individual differences in lymphoid cells, in terms of how they perceive and respond to an antigenic stimulus (see above). In the protein carrier itself, antigenic heterogeneity can arise from contamination, isosomal variation in protein structure, polymerization, and partial degradation, either in vitro or in vivo. Antigen heterogeneity can also occur when molecules of hapten become substituted on different functional amino acids or different sites on the protein, or it can occur from chemical contaminants of the hapten present de novo or formed during conjugation, dialysis, storage, or metabolic degradation in vivo. Conceivably, even the microheterogeneity created by the partial burying of hydrophobic haptenic groups in internal areas of the protein is a factor in the heterogeneous antibody response (Singer, 1964). Most studies indicate that even when the hapten on the immunizing antigen is substituted at a single site on a completely homogeneous protein, a heterogenous antibody results (Eisen et al., 1964; Little and Counts, 1969). However, examples are known in which a much more homogenous antibody has been obtained by using this strategy, as shown by hapten binding or gel electrophoresis studies of L-chain heterogeneity (Brenneman and Singer, 1968; Keck et al., 1973). Essentially homogeneous antibodies have also been obtained by immunization with carbohydrate antigens in bacterial cell walls (Krause, 1970) and even with selected proteins (Mamet-Bradley, 1966), although this situation is unusual.

Even though random coupling of a hapten to a protein favors a heterogeneous antibody response, this process may increase the possibility of obtaining a subpopulation of antibodies with desirable binding characteristics (see below). Therefore special efforts to immunize with a homogenous hapten-protein conjugate obtained by careful control of the conjugation reaction or fractionation of heterogeneous conjugate mixtures appear to be unnecessary and may even be undesirable.

Both small and large haptens induce heterogeneous antibody responses. Fractionation of antisera to large determinants usually reveals a spectrum of antibodies with specificities for various-sized segments of the immunogen. The antibody fraction or antiserum with the broadest area of recognition does not necessarily have an especially high affinity for the complete immunogen because it may be less well adapted to the immunodominant region. This fact can be readily appreciated by comparing the affinities of the two antitetrapeptide antibodies in Table 4.3 for DNP-lysine and the homologous DNP-tetrapeptide. These antibodies were obtained by using an identical immunization procedure on two different rabbits (Parker et al., 1966).

CHARGE AND PH EFFECTS ON BINDING

The binding of antibody to charged ligands is markedly influenced by pH and ionic strength (Pressman and Grossberg, 1968). Thus antibodies to p-azobenzoate, which has a single negative charge on its carboxylate groups at neutral pH, bind the hapten very poorly at pH 2. At this pH, the hapten carboxylate group is largely in the form of the free acid ($pK_a = 3.6$). An increase in ionic strength also reduces the binding of charged haptens, presumably because of the reciprocal relationship between the efficiency of transmission of charge through a liquid medium over short distances and the dielectric constant of the solvent. As a rule, the introduction of an extraneously charged group (not represented on the immunizing hapten) considerably decreases binding, especially if it is located in or near the immunodominant portion of the molecule. When the hapten is uncharged, changes in pH or ionic strength exert less of an effect on binding (Velick et al., 1960), but the binding may be more susceptible to organic solvents, such as dimethylformamide or dioxane, presumably due to interference with hydrophobic bond formation (Hurwitz et al., 1965) (see below).

STERIC HINDRANCE

Bulky substituents that are not represented on the immunizing hapten diminish binding (steric hindrance). This occurrence may be due to an interpenetration of electron clouds that results in an inability of the antibody-combining site to position the hapten properly and prevents the juxtaposition of interacting groups on the hapten and the antibody as required for optimization of binding. Substituents may also produce inductive or resonance effects on polarizability, thus altering the ionization of functional groups on the hapten and resulting in altered binding. Steric hindrance depends to a considerable extent on the nature and location of the substituent and the particular haptenic system involved. Antibodies appear to fit especially tightly around negatively charged functional groups, such as —COO⁻, and replacement by another group of the same charge may result in almost total loss of binding. When antibodies are prepared to diphenyl determinants, steric hindrance is much greater for bulky substituents on the distal (immunodominant) phenyl ring than for the same substitutent on the proximal ring (Pressman and Grossberg, 1968). This finding would seem to indicate that the antibody fits much more closely around the distal segment, in accordance with the greater contribution of this portion of the molecule to binding.

The Structural Basis for Antibody Specificity

STUDIES ON THE ROLE OF PRIMARY AMINO ACID SEQUENCE IN ANTIBODY SPECIFICITY

With the latest technical and conceptual advances in protein chemistry, it has been possible to elucidate partially the structural basis for antibody specificity. It has been shown that antibody molecules contain variable and constant regions in their H and L chains. There is now ample evidence that antibody specificity depends on the primary amino acid sequence in the variable regions of these chains. It is possible to largely or completely unfold intact antibody molecules or Fab fragments by reducing the disulfide bonds and disrupting the noncovalent bonds with unfolding reagents. As a result of the unfolding process, antigen binding is lost. After altered antibody molecules have been allowed to refold and reoxidize, substantial amounts of antigen-binding activity can be recovered (Haber, 1964; Whitney and Tanford, 1965; Freedman and Sela, 1966). The precise configuration of the antibody-binding site has only been partially elucidated, but it is presumed to be a cavity in which multiple amino acid residues from paired H and L chains establish close contact with the antigen.

The concept that there is structural complementarity between the antibody-combining region and antigen has been directly verified in the case of antibodies to charged haptens. Koshland and Englberger (1963) doubly immunized rabbits with the positively charged hapten, *p*-azotrimethylaminophenyl, and the negatively charged hapten, p-azobenzenearso-nate. The antibodies were purified and compared in regard to amino acid composition. Antibodies to the positively charged hapten had two more residues of glutamic acid and four more residues of aspartic acid (six extra negative charges), whereas antibodies to the negatively charged hapten had two more residues of arginine (two extra positive charges). The two antibodies were strikingly similar in their composition of other amino acids, with the exception of leucine and isoleucine. It was later shown that similar alterations in charged amino acids were demonstrable in Fab regions of the antibodies and that the changes were independent of allotypic specificity and immunoglobulin class (Koshland et al., 1969). Thus antibodies specific for these two charged haptens contain an increased number of oppositely charged amino acid residues. Presumably at least one of the oppositely charged residues is in the combining region, where it can undergo a short-range electrostatic interaction with hapten.

REVERSIBLE CHEMICAL MODIFICATION STUDIES

Confirmation of ionic complementarity of amino acids in the site has been obtained in chemical modification studies that demonstrated that when the putative, functional amino acid residue in the site is chemically blocked and then unblocked, the expected loss and restoration of hapten binding occur. Thus when rabbit antibody to the positively charged tri-methylphenylammonium group was treated with diazoacetamide, which esterifies negatively charged carboxyl groups, much of the binding activity was lost (Pressman and Grossberg, 1968). Following saponification of the ester groups at pH 11, a portion of the lost binding activity was re-covered. Esterification with diazoacetamide in the presence of homologous hapten resulted in diminished inactivation, presumably because a critical carboxyl group in the antibody-combining site was prevented from react-ing with the reagent. Similar results have been obtained following maleyla-tion and demaleylation of amino groups in antibenzenearsonate antibody (Freedman et al., 1968). There is little doubt that antibodies to other charged determinants are also programmed to contain appropriately charged amino acids in their combining regions. Indeed, the flexibility of the immune response is such that, following immunization with p-azo-benzenearsonate—a molecule that exists in mono- and dianionic forms at neutral pH—antibodies with specificities for each of the two charged states can be formed (Kreiter and Pressman, 1964).

TYPES OF BINDING FORCES INVOLVED IN ANTIBODY-HAPTEN INTERACTIONS

Even in antibody-hapten interactions involving charged determinants, it is certain that the bond that is formed requires additional binding forces

rather than electrostatic binding energy alone. Thus in antibodies to the
p-azobenzenearsonate group

$$—N—N—\langle O \rangle—AsO_3^= \quad \text{or} \quad —N—N—\langle O \rangle—AsO_3^-$$

the charged arsonate group contributes less to the total binding energy
than the benzene ring itself. Nonetheless, the contribution of the charged
group is sufficiently great that when the charge is lost, binding is greatly
diminished. Forces that contribute to antibody-hapten interactions probably include ionic bonds, hydrogen bonds, hydrophobic bonds, charge-
transfer bonds, and van der Waal's forces. The importance of hydrophobic
forces in the binding of uncharged haptens can be inferred from studies
with antibodies to the fluorescent 5-dimethylaminonaphthalene-l-lysyl
(DNS) group (Parker et al., 1966; Parker et al., 1967a, 1967b). The
antibody-bound hapten (ϵ-DNS-lysine) undergoes a marked increase in
fluorescence quantum yield and marked blue shift in the emission maximum, closely simulating the changes obtained when the free hapten is
dissolved in nonpolar organic solvents. Thus the microenvironment of the
hapten in the antibody-combining site appears to simulate a solvent of
low dielectric constant. Presumably the high maximal affinity obtainable
with antibody-hapten interactions involving hydrophobic determinants is
a reflection of the relatively large change in free energy when multiple
hydrophobic interactions occur. But the binding is not solely hydrophobic
in character, for if it were, the stability of the antibody-hapten complex
should be unaffected or even increased with increasing temperature,
whereas the converse is observed. Similar observations have been made
with 2,4-dinitrophenyl and p-iodoacetylaminobenzeneazohippurate haptens,
where the direction and magnitude changes in enthalpy and entropy argue
against a pure hydrophobic interaction (Eisen and Siskind, 1964; Fujio
and Karush, 1966; Parker et al., 1967a). Attempts to implicate hydrogen
bonding as the dominant binding force in antibody-hapten interactions
encounter much the same difficulties. In the DNP system some of the
binding energy may be supplied by a charge-transfer interaction between
electron-seeking DNP groups and a tryptophan residue in the antibody-
combining region (Little and Eisen, 1967). Of the various amino acids
present in proteins, tryptophan is best able to serve as an electron donor.
In any event, it seems highly likely that the bond that is formed between
hapten and antibody represents a summation of a number of different
binding forces, the exact pattern depending on the particular hapten and
antibody (Eisen, 1966). It follows that the greater the number and
magnitude of the contributing forces, the greater the stability of the bond.
As a further corollary, if only a portion of the haptenic determinant to
which the antibody is adapted is available for binding, the strength of the
interaction will be diminished, thus explaining the decrease in DNP-ligand
binding by anti-DNP-lysyl antibodies as the number of carbons attached

to the DNP group is decreased from 5 to 0 (Fig. 4.1). In a given antibody-hapten system the relative contributions by ionic, hydrophobic, and hydrogen bonds will help determine how changes in pH, ionic strength, temperature, and the dielectric constant influence the antibody-hapten interaction. For example, as already discussed, ionic interactions are affected by changes in pH and ionic strength, whereas hydrophobic interactions are more susceptible to changes in the dielectric properties of the medium. Hydrogen-bond stability decreases with increasing temperature, but the strength of a hydrophobic bond is unchanged or slightly increased. From a knowledge of the structural properties of the hapten, reasonable predictions can be made as to how binding might be optimized. However, even if a complete profile of the various binding forces involved in the interaction of antibody with hapten were available (which it is not), some empiricism would be needed, since alterations in the temperature and composition of the medium could also influence antibody or hapten structure, thereby complicating the analysis.

Protein Specificity

Types of Antigenic Determinants on Proteins

As a rule, antibody specificity to proteins and other macromolecules seems to be determined relatively early in the immune response and is directed in large measure toward the intact macromolecule rather than its degradation fragments. Three general types of antigenic sites have been recognized: (a) *sequential determinants* composed of linear oligopeptides, oligosaccharides, or oligonucleotides in which primary structure is recognized; (b) *conformational determinants* involving folded or cross-linked areas in which secondary, tertiary, or even quaternary structure is recognized; and (c) *haptenic determinants* in which chemically altered amino acids, monosaccharides, or mononucleotides are recognized (e.g., triiodothyronine in thyroglobulin).

Limitations in the Size of the Antibody-combining Site

All three types of determinants involve a limited cross-sectional area of the immunizing macromolecule. Estimates of the maximal area of recognition of an antibody for a sequential antigenic determinant are available from immunological studies with antibodies to linear polymers of alanine and glucose. In the case of antibodies to polyalanine (obtained by immunization with polyalanine attached to a protein carrier), competitive inhibition studies indicated that the pentamer (ala)$_5$ inhibited as well or better than the hexamer (ala)$_6$ (Sage et al., 1964). The dimensions of the (ala)$_5$ molecule were calculated to be 25 × 11 × 6 A (assuming an extended configuration). This would correspond to a contact area on the antibody site of roughly 2,000 Å² if the oligopeptide is telescoped into a cylindrical antibody-combining site or 700 Å² in the event of binding to a shallow groove on the surface of the antibody molecule with a portion of the bound oligopeptide segment projecting above the surface of the antibody. Kabat had earlier made similar studies of the size of the antibody-combining site in antibodies to dextran (a glucose polymer) and concluded that the hexasaccharide was the best inhibitor (Kabat, 1954). The hexasaccharide would be a determinant of very similar size to pentaalanine (again 2,000 or 700 Å², depending on whether a deep or a shallow antibody-combining site is visualized). Estimates of the size of antigenic determinants in linear oligopeptides of silk fibroin (Cebra, 1961), poly-α-D-glutamic acid (Goodman et al., 1968), and α-DNP-oligolysines (David and Schlossman, 1968) are a little larger (6 to 10 amino acid residues) but, clearly, still fall within the realm of determinants of restricted size. The type of data leading to this conclusion is illustrated for silk fibroin in Fig. 4.3. These observations with model

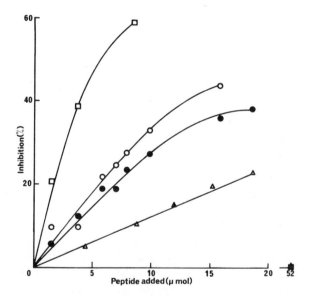

Fig. 4.3. Comparison of the capacities of a homologous series of peptides of increasing size to inhibit the precipitation of soluble silk fibroin by an antiserum from a rabbit immunized with soluble fibroin absorbed to blood charcoal; ■, Gly-L-Ala; ▲, Gly [Gly, Val] Tyr; △, Gly [Gly, Ala] Tyr; ●, Gly [Gly$_3$, Ala$_2$, Val] Tyr; o, Gly [Gly$_3$, Ala$_3$] Tyr and □, a mixture of (Gly [Gly$_3$, Ala$_3$] Tyr) and (Gly [Gly, Ala] Tyr) (Gly [Gly$_3$, Ala$_2$, Val] Tyr), etc. (i.e., dodecapeptides). Increasing amounts of peptide were incubated with a constant volume of antiserum and then with a standard amount of antigen. The inhibition (%) represents the decrease in amount of precipitate formed in the presence of peptide. (Taken from J. J. Cebra. 1961. J. Immunol. 86:205–214.)

polyaminoacid and polysaccharide determinants clearly indicate the ability of animals to form antibodies to linear determinants and give some notion of the area of recognition involved.

Studies with model synthetic polypeptides have also been useful in helping develop the concept of conformational determinants. Gill and his colleagues (1965) have immunized animals with polypeptides cross linked in various ways and showed that antibodies may be formed to determinants in areas of linkage between two chains. Studies with antibodies to synthetic polymers containing repeating units of Pro-Gly-Pro, which exists in solution in the form of a triple helix, indicate the feasibility of obtaining antibodies to polypeptide sequences in a helical configuration as well as to the random-coil structures (Sela et al., 1967). These antibodies have affinity for collagen from various sources that also form triple-stranded helixes. An ability to recognize tertiary structure is also indicated in studies with polyamino acids containing Tyr-Ala-Glu sequences. Antibodies to sequences of Tyr-Ala-Glu in a random-coil configuration (attached through poly-D, L-alanine to a polylysine backbone) cross-react poorly or not at all with antibodies to Tyr-Ala-Glu polymers in an α-helical configuration (Sela et al., 1967).

Studies of the Antigenic Specificity of Proteins

Much of our knowledge of the various types of antigenic determinants on proteins comes from studies with proteins of defined amino acid sequence and three-dimensional structure (lysozyme, myoglobulin, ribonuclease, and chymotrypsin). The importance of tertiary structure is evident from the studies of Brown and his colleagues (1959) with native and oxidized ribonuclease (RNase). Antibodies to native RNase, which contains four disulfide bonds, did not react with performic acid-oxidized RNase, which is in a random-coil configuration but has the same amino acid sequence as the unaltered enzyme (except at oxidized half-cystine residues). When performic acid-oxidized RNase was used as the immunogen, antibodies with a different specificity were obtained, and two polypeptide sequences (residues 38–61 and 105–124) from different regions of the enzyme were shown to inhibit binding (Brown, 1962). Thus immunization with the native enzyme did not produce antibodies to sequential determinants, whereas immunization with the oxidized enzyme did. Similar results have been obtained with antibodies to native bovine and human serum albumin, apomyoglobulin, and flagellin, where antigenic reactivity was greatly reduced when the proteins were degraded to polypeptide units having molecular weights of 5,000 or below (Porter, 1957; Crumpton and Wilkinson, 1965, Ada et al., 1967). For example, the most active chymotryptic peptide of apomyoglobulin inhibited precipitation of the intact protein by antibody by only 15%, and the digest as a whole was only modestly inhibitory (Crumpton and Wilkinson, 1965). On the other hand, larger fragments of apomyoglobulin, produced by cyanogen bromide cleavage at the two methionine residues of the molecule, had a total reactivity equal to that of the intact molecule (Atassi and Saplin, 1968). Thus ribonuclease, serum albumins, apomyoglobulin, and flagellin appear to be proteins in which the antigenic determinants are largely of the conformational type. Interestingly, when the N-terminal cyanogen bromide fragment (1–55) was used as the immunogen, antibodies with a new specificity were formed, as evidenced by much more effective precipitation of fragment (1–55) than intact myoglobulin (Fig. 4.4).

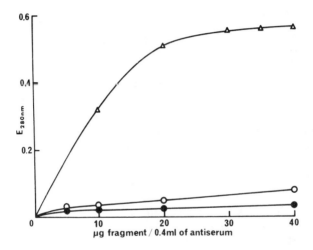

Fig. 4.4. Precipitation of the N-terminal cyanogen bromide fragment (residues 1–55) of sperm whale myoglobin (△), the native protein (●, metmyoglobin), and apomyoglobin (o) by an antiserum against the fragment. (Taken from M. J. Crumpton. 1974. In M. Sela (Ed.). The Antigens. Vol. II. Academic Press, New York. pp. 1–78.)

A somewhat different picture emerged in studies with egg-white lysozyme. Arnon and Sela (1969) isolated a peptide that contained residues 64 to 83 of the enzyme. When the peptide was in the form of a loop (joined by one-half cystines at residues 64 and 80), it reacted with antibodies to native lysozyme, whereas the open-chain peptide (obtained by reduction of the disulfide bond) was unreactive, thus indicating the existence of a conformational determinant. On the other hand, Thompson and Levy (1970), working with a linear synthetic polypeptide containing residues 74 to 83 (the C-terminal portion of Arnon and Sela's peptide) and a different antilysozymal antibody, were able to show considerable binding of the peptide to antibody. Taking the results of the two studies together, it would appear that the same area of the native lysozyme molecule can serve either as a sequential or a conformational determinant, depending on the antiserum. Further evidence for sequential determinants on native lysozyme comes from the work of Young and Leon (1970), who showed that the N-terminal peptide 1–12 was immunologically reactive with antibodies to the native protein.

The role of sequential determinants in the protein coat of tobacco mosaic virus (TMVP) is even more striking. This protein has only one major antigenic determinant representing residues 93 to 112 at the C-terminal end of the molecule (Benjamini et al., 1968). Essentially all the anti-TMVP antibody can be bound by the isolated 93–112 eicosapeptide.

Factors in Antibody Formation and Reactivity to
Protein Antigens

STERIC ACCESSIBILITY

Regardless of whether an antigenic determinant on a protein is sequential or confirmational, it is likely to be in an area of the molecule where it is sterically accessible to antibody. It has been known since the early 1960s, from the studies of Sela and his colleagues with antibodies to model multichain polyamino acids, that although the antigenic determinant need not necessarily be at the end of a peptide chain, it cannot be hidden in the interior of the molecule (Katchalski et al., 1964) (Fig. 4.5). Thus immunization to polytyrosyl determinants was possible with molecules in which poly-D, L-alanyl side chains attached to a poly-L-lysine backbone were elongated with peptides containing tyrosine residues. No antibody

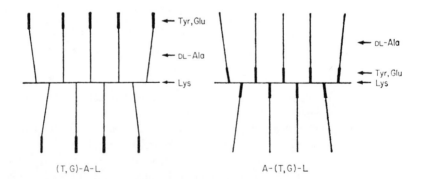

Fig. 4.5. Schematic diagram of a multichain copolymer with tyrosine (T) and glutamic acid (G) residues attached to multipoly-DL-alanyl poly-L-lysine, (T,G)-A-L, and of one with tyrosine and glutamic acid attached directly to the lysine backbone and then elongated with alanine, A-(T,G)-L. (Taken from M. Sela. 1962. *In* M. A. Stahman (Ed.). Polyamino acids, polypeptides and proteins. University of Wisconsin Press, Madison. p. 353.)

response was obtained when tyrosine-containing peptides were attached directly to the polymeric backbone and then covered with poly-D, L-alanine, even though the molecules resembled their immunogenic counterparts in terms of size, shape, and overall amino acid composition. But when alanine was added to the polymeric backbone, so that the side chains were spaced at less-frequent intervals, immunogenicity to internally located polytyrosyl residues was restored. Evidently the reduction in frequency of side chains permitted the tyrosine-containing peptides to gain access to cell receptors and trigger a response.

The importance of steric accessibility in immunization with intact proteins was initially shown in the studies of Crumpton and Wilkinson (1965) with myoglobulin, where it was found that antigenically active regions were likely to be at the ends or corners of the molecule. This finding is not surprising when the three-dimensional structure of the molecule is considered (Fig. 4.6). A similar conclusion has been reached in immunological studies

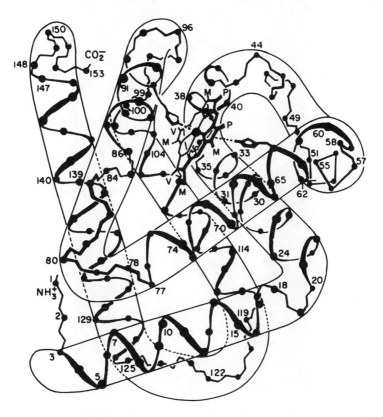

Fig. 4.6. A two-dimensional representation of the conformation of a molecule of sperm whale metmyoglobin. The amino acid residues are arranged in eight helical segments separated by nonhelical regions. (Taken from R. E. Dickerson. 1964. In H. Neurath (Ed.). The Proteins. Vol. II. Academic Press, New York. pp. 603–768.)

with tobacco mosaic virus (TMV). The three-dimensional structures of TMV is known to consist of an RNA core with 2,130 identical, closely packed polypeptide units projecting out from the core and with the C-terminal end of the molecule in the penultimate position (Fig. 4.7). Immunization with the intact virion regularly produces antibodies that are reactive with the C-terminal hexapeptide of the virus (residues 153–158) (Anderer and Schlumberger, 1965; Benjamini et al., 1965), the area of the TMV unit most accessible to antibody.

The importance of steric availability in immunogenicity is easily understood at the cellular level if a model for the immune response is chosen in which activation of antigen-sensitive cells take place at the cell surface. If it is assumed that activation requires a critical number of antigen molecules attached to a cell over a sustained period of time, this process

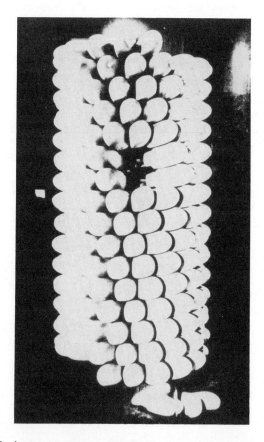

Fig. 4.7. Model of subunit arrangement in TMV based on X-ray scattering data. The virus consists of an RNA core and 2,130 identical polypeptide units in its protein coat. (Taken from H. Fraenkel-Conrat. 1965. In H. Neurath (Ed.). The Proteins. Vol. III. Academic Press, New York. pp. 99–151.)

is most likely to occur if the antigenic determinant involved is already present in the native protein (e.g., metabolic processing of the antigen is not required) and can bind to the cell without undergoing a major conformational change (e.g., binding does not require a large activation energy).

In addition to antibody formation to surface determinants on proteins, there is evidence that antibody formation can occur to "internal" antigenic determinants created or unmasked during denaturation or enzymatic degradation of the immunogen in vivo (Ishizaka et al., 1960). Although such formation increases the complexity of the immune response, for immunoassay purposes, the presence of antibodies to internal determinants is not likely to complicate the analysis, provided that the antigen marker itself is undegraded and antibodies to the internal determinants do not recognize the native protein (see below).

ANTIGENIC FOREIGNESS

Considering the flexibility of the immune system, we would assume that any sterically available area on the surface of a protein is potentially immunogenic. But when animals are immunized with sizable proteins from other mammalian species, a restricted immune response is obtained. For example, bovine serum albumin (BSA; molecular weight 70,000) ordinarily has a maximal valence of 5–6, as judged by the number of antibody molecules that can be attached to the protein in far antibody excess. The limitation in the number of demonstrable antigenic sites is partially explained by limitations in the total surface area available for binding, resulting in steric hindrance to the simultaneous binding of multiple antibody molecules to the same molecule of antigen. Another factor is the considerable degree of structural homology among serum albumins in different mammalian species. When immunization is attempted in a background of immunological tolerance, only the portions of the immunogen that are truly foreign to the host will induce a response. Yalow has suggested that differences in degree of foreignness may explain why guinea pigs frequently develop a better antibody response to insulin and several other human polypeptide hormones than rabbits (Yalow and Berson, 1971). But even if a protein that is unique to invertebrates is used for immunization, there is the possibility of an unrecognized partial homology, with a protein in the animal undergoing immunization, thus altering the response.

Because of the importance of foreignness in immunogenicity, if the degree of structural homology between the immunogen and the corresponding endogenous protein in various mammalian and avian species is known, a rational choice as to which species to immunize may be possible. However, it is important to emphasize that antigenic cross-reactivity is not a linear function of differences in amino acid composition per se. Studies with myoglobulin and cytochrome c indicate that many amino acid replacements or deletions have little or no effect on antigenic reactivity, whereas other, seemingly small changes produce major effects. A good example is the antigenic distinction made between human and monkey cytochrome c with rabbit anticytochrome c antibodies (Nisonoff et al., 1970). Human and monkey cytochrome c's differ only at residues 58 (isoleucine and threonine, respectively); yet as many as 40% of the antihuman cytochrome c antibodies fail to bind with the monkey protein. Obviously the isoleucine residue in the human cytochrome is a key residue in a major antigenic area of the protein. Interestingly, when monkey cytochrome c is the immunogen, the rabbit antibodies fail to distinguish between the human and monkey protein. Rabbits and monkeys both contain threonine at residue 58, and no antibodies are obtained to this region of the protein. Since this is the only area in which human and monkey cytochrome c differ in their primary structure, the antibodies react identically with the two proteins. The experience with cytochrome c indicates the danger in attempting to use immunologic cross-reactivity to discern phylogenetic relationships. This point is further illustrated when the extent of immunological cross-reactivity and degree of difference in amino acid sequence are expressed graphically for a variety of globular proteins (Fig. 4.8). The lesson in terms of immunoassay development is that if initial immunization attempts are unrewarding, there may be merit in trying new species. The principle of utilizing a species as phylogenetically removed as possible was exploited by Reiss and Canterbury (1969), who immunized chickens with bovine parathyroid hormone (BPTH) and obtained antibodies with relatively high cross-reactivity for human PTH. Antibodies produced in mammals were less satisfactory.

ANTIGENIC COMPETITION

Another factor affecting the diversity of antibodies produced to a foreign protein is antigenic competition. When an immunogen contains both strong and weak antigenic determinants, the initial response is likely to involve the strong determinants. As immunization is continued over a period of several months, the diversity of antibodies produced increases and antibodies that are specific for the weak determinants can be demonstrated. This situation is exemplified by the response to rat-skin collagen in rabbits. Collagen contain two types of polypeptide chains, α-1 and α-2. Generally the immune response is directed toward sequential determinants in the C- and N-terminal ends of these chains, although antibodies may also be formed to internal antigenic determinants or to the triple helical

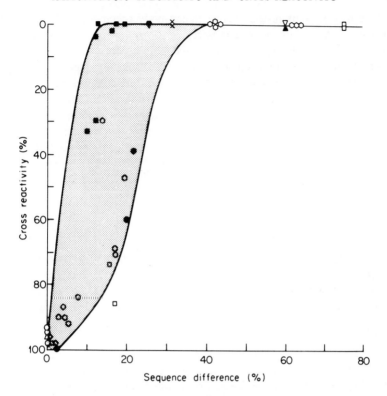

Fig. 4.8. Correlation between immunologic cross-reactivity and difference in amino acid sequence for various globular protein families. Cross-reactivity was determined either by microcomplement fixation or by quantitative precipitation: alkaline phosphatase (⊗), carbonic anhydrase (△), growth hormone-placental lactogen (●), ferredoxin (▼), penicillinase (▲), trypsin-chymotrypsin (▽), pancreatice ribonuclease (●), β-lactoglobulin (◇), subtilisin (X), RNA phage coat protein (□); hemoglobin (0), myoglobin (■), and lysozyme (◯). The shaded area indicates the range of sequence differences over which cross-reactivity generally occurs. (Taken from E. M. Prager, and A. C. Wilson. 1971. J. Biol. Chem. 246:7010–7017.)

configuration of assembled collagen (see above) (Timpl et al., 1972). During the early phases of immunization, antibodies directed largely or entirely toward the C-terminal ends of the α-1 and α-2 chains of the molecule are produced. Later in the response, antibodies directed toward the N-terminal ends of the α-1 and α-2 chains appear, and the response to the C-terminal end of the α-1 chain diminishes. The time-dependent change in antibody specificity is not overridden by the use of high doses of antigen. Thus by lengthening the time after which the antiserum is harvested, not only are new antibody specificities appearing, but there may be a partial dropping out of specificities present previously as well. Obviously these changes in immunological specificity could have an important influence on immunoassay sensitivity and cross-reactivity.

One way to explain the change in antibody specificity with time is by assuming that initially only cells with receptors for the stronger determinants take up the antigen. After antibodies are formed, the strong determinants become complexed by antibody and masked, thereby permitting an immune response to weak determinants on the same molecule. Another possibility is that highly immunogenic determinants aid in the response to weak determinants in much the same way that an immunogenic protein carrier amplifies the response to simple chemical determinants. According to this view, the delay in obtaining antibodies to secondary determinants is the time required for the immunodominant determinants to generate the necessary level of cellular binding and immunologic inflamation to permit an additional response.

GENETIC RESPONSIVENESS

In addition to the role of three-dimensional structure and foreigness in immune responsiveness, the genetic makeup of the animal has an important influence on the quantity and quality of the antibodies produced. There are marked differences between highly inbred strains of guinea pigs or mice in their responses to relatively simple antigens, such as the synthetic polyamino acids. Thus two mouse strains immunized with the same polypeptide antigen may have a hundredfold or greater differences in their serum antibody titers. Careful genetic studies have revealed that the genes controlling immune responsiveness (Ir genes) are inhibited as a Mendelian-dominant characteristic and are closely linked to genes determining the major histocompatibility antigens (McDevitt and Benaceraff, 1969). The Ir genes also influence immune responsiveness to naturally occurring polypeptides and proteins and to haptens, although the magnitude of the effect is not as great as with simple polypeptides (Sobey and Adams, 1961).

Genetic factors influence antibody specificity as well as antibody quantity. Arquilla and Finn (1965) compared the immune response to bovine insulin in two inbred guinea pig strains. Although both strains produced antiinsulin antibodies, it could be shown by competitive binding that the regions of the insulin molecule involved in antibody binding were not the same in the two strains. Presumably the average affinities of the antibodies for insulin also differed, although this distinction was not directly demonstrated. From these and other studies it is evident that antigenic areas of protein are not fixed but vary, depending on the species and even on the individual animal immunized. The quantity of immunogen required to produce an optimal response and the mode of evolution of the response also vary in different animal strains.

Studies in inbred animals help to answer a question that is frequently raised by investigators interested in developing immunoassays: Is there a single animal species or strain that would be a superior antibody producer regardless of the antigen? The answer is an unequivocal no. In both guinea pigs and mice, an inbred strain that responds with exceptional vigor to a given polypeptide antigen may respond poorly or not at all to another, not too dissimilar antigen. For any given antigen, the strain of animals with the most favorable response characteriistic would have to be identified empirically, but once this step had been accomplished, that strain could be used for all subsequent immunizations. Unfortunately, a wide assortment of highly inbred animals is not available except in mice, and so outbred animals must be used. Even without inbred animals, the problem of individual variation in responsiveness can be solved by breeding male and female animals having favorable immune response characteristics. Because immune response patterns seem to be inherited as Mendelian-dominant characteristics, all the progeny could then be expected to respond in the desired way. Fortunately, most immunoassay procedures do not require strenuous effects to identify suitable antiserum producers. In general, the immunization of 8 or 10 outbred rabbits will provide at least several antisera that are satisfactory for assay.

Immunologic Cross-reactivity Between Proteins

Antigenic cross-reactivity can be a major limiting factor in the usefulness of immunological measurements. It is therefore important to consider the different types of immunological cross-reactivity and how they may be circumvented or minimized.

PROTEINS THAT CONTAIN SIMILAR (OR IDENTICAL) AS WELL AS DISSIMILAR DETERMINANTS

Multichain proteins or polypeptides. One type of immunological cross-reactivity occurs with multichain proteins having one chain that is very similar or identical and another that is dissimilar. This situation is seen with follicle-stimulating hormone (FSH), thyroid-stimulating hormone (TSH), human chorionic gonadotrophin (HCG), and luteinizing hormone (LH), which are sizable proteins with different β chains and very similar α chains (Burr et al., 1969; Grant and Butt, 1970; Midgley et al., 1971). The differing biologic activities of these proteins are based on their different β chains. The most successful approach to cross-reactivity has been to immunize many animals, select the most specific antisera, and absorb with one or more of the cross-reacting antigens. Midgley et al. (1971) have suggested that heterologous FSH reagents may be used to obtain reagents for determining human FSH based on the empirical observation that cross-reactivity is sometimes decreased with a heterologous marker or immunizing antigen.

Immunologic cross-reactivity between proteins produced in different species can also be helpful in the development of immunoassays for human proteins that are not available in sufficient quantities for immunization. Thus porcine insulin, which differs from human insulin only at the 30 position of the β chain, can be used both as an immunogen and as a radioactive marker in the measurement of human insulin (Yalow and Berson, 1971). Indeed, with some antisera, the human and porcine hormones react identically. Sometimes the antibodies react so much better with the immunizing protein than with the protein under study that still another species must be used as a source for the marker protein. The result is to reduce the affinity of the antibody for the marker, thereby making the human protein better able to compete. Thus human prolactin does not displace ^{125}I ovine prolactin from guinea pig-antiovine prolactin antibody, but a sensitive curve is obtained with an ^{125}I porcine prolactin marker (Jacobs et al., 1972).

The development of heterologous immunoassays is not possible with every protein. Human TSH, for example, apparently exhibits so little structural similarity to TSH in other species that useful levels of immunologic cross-reactivity are not obtained, even though there is no species specificity in the biological reactivity of TSH (Utiger, 1974).

Single-chain proteins or polypeptides. Immunological cross-reactivity can also occur between single-chain proteins that have substantial areas of homology. This point is exemplified by adrenocorticotrophic hormones (ACTH) and α and β melanotrophic hormones (MSH), which have common amino acid sequences in the N-terminal portion of their molecules and overlapping biological and immunological reactivities. Human ACTH is a straight-chain polypeptide that contains 39 acid residues. Its biological activity is contained in its first 24 amino acids (ACTH, α^{1-24}). Human α-MSH is an Nα-acetylated polypeptide composed of the first 13 N-terminal amino acids of ACTH; human β-MSH has 22 amino acids, 7 of which are common with ACTH and α-MSH (residues 2 to 8). Not surprisingly, then, ACTH and α-MSH have greater immunologic cross-reactivity for one another than for B-MSH. The N-terminal portion of ACTH is also the region of the molecule that is the most homologous in different species, whereas the C-terminal areas in different ACTHs are quite dissimilar, creating the theoretical possibility of obtaining anti-ACTH antibodies that are largely species specific (antibodies to the C-terminal end of the molecule) or that have marked cross-reactivity (antibodies to the N-terminal end of the molecule). Experiments have verified this feature. Antibodies to whole human ACTH are normally directed primarily toward the 15 amino acids at the C-terminal end of the molecule, and there is little or no cross-reactivity with ACTHs from other species or with α- and B-MSH. But some anti-ACTH antisera have considerable specificity for various segments of the N-terminal or central portions of the molecule, and here the expected cross-reactivity is observed. Thus even as small a polypeptide as ACTH, which has only 39 amino acids, has several antigenic areas (Fig. 4.9); and depending on where the immunologic specificity of the antibody is directed, much or little antigenic cross-reactivity may be seen.

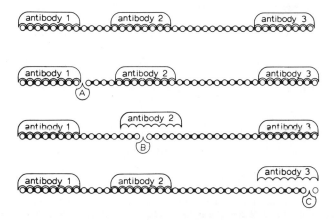

Fig. 4.9. Diagrammatic representation of the 39 amino acid chain of ACTH and its interaction with antibodies of three different specificities. Antibody 1 reacts with the 1–8 sequence, antibody 2 with the 13–20 sequence, and antibody 3 with the 32–39 sequence of amino acid residues. Three enzymes that cleave the ACTH molecule as indicated can be used to alter binding selectively, depending on which antibody is used. Enzyme A cleaves the 8–9 bond, enzyme B the 15–16 bond, and enzyme C the 38–39 peptide bond. (Taken from D. N. Orth. 1975. *In* B. W. O'Malley, and J. G. Hardman (Eds.). Methods in enzymology. Vol. 37. Academic Press, New York. pp. 22–38.)

Because of the presence of multiple antigenic areas on ACTH, it is possible to tailor-make antisera with the desired specificity characteristics. Since the N-terminal end of ACTH is the biologically active portion, most investigators have chosen to use antisera that recognize this portion of the molecule for immunoassay measurements. Doing so reduces the possibility that partially degraded molecules of ACTH that have lost their biological activity would be detected in the assay and reduces the necessity for using homologous ACTH as a marker and standard in the assay.

Antibodies to the N-terminal end of ACTH can be obtained by several methods. In addition to screening a number of antisera to whole ACTH in an attempt to identify a serum with N-terminal specificity, antisera to synthetic $α^{1-24}$ ACTH, porcine ACTH, or periodate-oxidized ACTH may be used. Examples of different radioimmunoassay inhibition curves with different antisera are given in Figs. 4.10, 4.11, and 4.12.

The feasibility of manipulating antigenic specificity and cross-reactivity in proteins or polypeptides by the degradation or synthesis of anti-

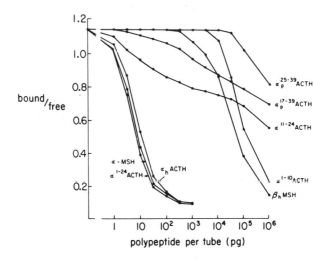

Fig. 4.10. Specificity of an antibody to the extreme N-terminal end of ACTH. The competitive binding curves generated by the addition of graded amounts of a variety of unlabeled ACTH and MSH analogs are shown. The antibody reacts fully with any polypeptide containing the 1–13 sequence of amino acids of ACTH. (Taken from D. N. Orth. 1974. *In* B. M. Jaffe, and H. R. Behrman (Eds.). Methods of hormone radioimmunoassay. Academic Press, New York. pp. 125–159.)

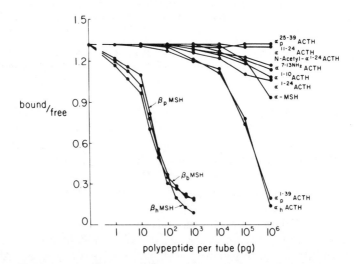

Fig. 4.11. Specificity of an antibody directed toward the C-terminal end of ACTH. This antibody reacts fully with any polypeptide containing the 25–39 sequence of human or porcine ACTH, which differ only in position 31. (Taken from D. N. Orth. 1974. *In* B. M. Jaffe, and H. R. Behrman (Eds.). Methods of hormone radioimmunoassay. Academic Press, New York. pp. 125–159.)

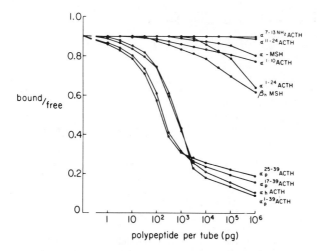

Fig. 4.12. Specificity of an antibody raised in a guinea pig to porcine β-MSH. β-hMSH was used as labeled tracer. Neither ACTH nor α-MSH reacts sufficiently with the antibody to present any problem in radioimmunoassay. (Taken from D. N. Orth. 1974. *In* B. M. Jaffe, and H. R. Behrman (Eds.). Methods of hormone radioimmunoassay. Academic Press, New York. pp. 125–159.)

genically active fragments is much greater for some antigens than for others. Parathyroid hormone (PTH) is similar to ACTH in having both species-specific and species cross-reactive regions. Immunoglobulins are particularly amenable to antigenic fractionation because of their susceptibility to enzymatic and chemical cleavage with formation of large functionally and structurally distinct antigenic fragments that retain their full immunologic reactivity. PTH and ACTH can also be manipulated in this way. The separation of multichain proteins into individual chains may or may not be associated with major losses of antigenic reactivity. Isolated α and β chains of FSH, TSH, and LH continue to react with antibodies to the intact proteins, but with the usual antiporcine or bovine insulin antisera, the isolated α and β chains of the two insulins lose essentially all their immunologic reactivity. Additional examples of immunologically cross-reacting proteins or polypeptides and the extremes of cross-reactivity that are possible are given in Table 4.4.

PROTEINS AND POLYPEPTIDES THAT UNDERGO
PROTEOLYTIC DEGRADATION

Another type of immunologic cross-reactivity is exhibited by different proteolytic species of proteins:

1. "Big hormones." A number of hormones are normally converted from high molecular weight precursors to the active hormone by proteolysis

Table 4.4

Examples of cross-reacting or polypeptide hormones occurring in human serum or tissue and the extremes of cross-reactivity that are possible.

	Molecular size (number of amino acid residues)	Area of homology	Relative immunoassay cross-reactivity	
			Maximal	Minimal
1. ACTH	39			
α-MSH	13	1–13 (same)	1.0	<0.00025 ‡
B-MSH	22	11–17 (4–10)	0.001	<0.0001
2. Growth H	190			
HCS	190	85%	–	0.0001
Prolactin	~195	<25%	0.1	<0.001
3. TSH	~196			
HCG	~168	α chain	0.25	<0.001
FSH	comparable	α chain	0.50	0.02
LH	~168	α chain	0.40	0.001
4. Gastrin	17			
CPZ	33	29–33 (13–17)	0.04	0.001
5. LVP	8			
AVP	8	1–6, 8 (same)	1.0	0.4
Oxytocin	8	1–2, 4–6, 8 (same)	0.0004	<0.0001
6. AGT I	10			
AGT II	8	1–8 (same)	1.0	<0.001
7. Secretin	27			
Glucagon †	29	1–2, 4–8, 11 (same) 15–16, 18, 20 26	–	<0.0001 †

* The $\sim$ sign indicates either that different results have been obtained in different laboratories or that the amino acid sequence is not fully known. The number in ( ) refers to the area of homology on the polypeptide to which it is being compared.* Cross-reactivity is measured in the homologous reference immunoassay system (e.g., the data given for α-MSH cross-reactivity is based on its inhibitory activity relative to ACTH in the ACTH anti-ACTH system). Unless otherwise specified, the data are for the human hormones. AGT is angiotensin; LVP and AVP are lysine and arginnine vasopressin.

† Note that glucagon apparently fails to cross-react with antisecretin antibody despite the extensive structural homology between the two polypeptides. Presumably their three-dimensional structures are different (Boden, 1974).

‡ The marked differences in cross-reactivity seen with some of the antigens are primarily due to deliberate attempts to minimize cross-reactivity (antiserum selection, absorption, use of cross-reacting antigens or antigen fragments for immunization or radiolabeling; see Chapter 11).

before leaving the cell. Not infrequently, the precursor escapes into the venous system, creating a circulating, high molecular weight form of the hormone in addition to the active hormone itself (Steiner et al., 1968). Hormones that circulate in a high molecular form include insulin, parathormone (PTH), gastrin, glucagon, growth hormone, vasopressin, and ACTH. These "big hormones" cross-react immunologically with antibodies to the usual molecular form of the hormone, although the level of immunological reactivity is often less than might be expected on either a weight or a molar basis.

2. Immunologic cross-reactivity is also exhibited between such proteins as fibrinogen and fibrin, the product formed when fibrinogen undergoes enzymatic conversion in the circulation from an inactive to a biologically active form. After conversion to fibrin, the areas of the molecule that remain unaltered continue to react with antifibrinogen antibody, but with suitable antisera, immunologic discrimination should be possible in the areas of the molecule where conversion has taken place.

3. Large or small, biologically inactive peptide fragments split off from the parent molecule may continue to react immunologically with antibodies to the intact hormone. In immunoassay measurements of hormones and other biologically active macromolecules, this is a potential source of misinterpretation, since part of the total immunoreactivity may be due to inactive fragments.

4. Finally, new antigenic determinants may be created during enzymatic degradation. For example, sensitive immunoassays have been developed to small molecular weight peptides released when fibrinogen or fibrin is degraded by plasmin (fibrinogenolysis or fibrinolysis) (Plow and Edgington, 1973). The antigenic specificity expressed on the enzymatically generated peptides is masked on intact fibrinogen and fibrin. Although the conversion of fibrinogen to fibrin does not directly expose the peptide determinant, the immunochemical specificity of the peptide is altered, presumably because of a conformational change in a critical region of the fibrin molecule that changes the mode of cleavage by plasmin. This situation is reflected by a different slope in the immunoassay-dose inhibition curve (using rabbit antibody to fibrinogen cleavage peptide D and ^{125}I fibrinogen peptide D marker). The difference in immunochemical reactivity can be used to differentiate fibrinogenolysis from fibrinolysis. Changes in immunologic specificity can have also been to detect enzymatic alterations in other proteins including the third component of complement, pepsinogen, procarboxypeptidase (Barrett, 1965), and plasminogen (Rabiner et al., 1969); it seems likely this will be an important area for immunoassay application in the future.

PROTEINS THAT UNDERGO POLYMERIZATION

Polymerization may be associated with losses of immunological reactivity due to the masking of antigenically important areas of the protein. Thus as the degree of association of keyhole limpet hemocyanin in solution is increased, its total antigenic reactivity with antihemocyanin antibodies is decreased but can be recovered by reconverting the protein to its monomeric form (Weigle, 1964). In other situations in which there is diminished antigenic reactivity after aggregation, the very fact that polymerization has occurred may indicate that the protein has been denatured and has already lost immunologic reactivity. This may be the major explanation for the low immunological reactivity of large molecular weight subfractions of certain ^{125}I-labeled hormones (see below). On the other hand, the collection of multiple molecules of protein may create new antigenic determinants, giving the polymer a unique antigenic reactivity. This situation has been observed following polymerization of the H polypeptide chains on human IgG. The polymerized molecules assume a new antigenic specificity that is also present on heat or 6 M urea denatured IgG (Sela et al., 1967).

PROTEINS WITH COMMON HAPTENIC GROUPS

Proteins such as thyroglobulin that contain similar or identical haptenic groups (triiodothyronine and thyroxin) will cross-react immunologically even if they do not contain common protein determinants.

SPURIOUS CROSS-REACTIVITY

Immunological cross-reactivity is simulated when both the immunogen and the marker contain an immunologically unrelated contaminant.

SUMMARY

1. Antibodies to closely related haptens structurally exhibit clear-cut differences in primary amino acid sequence and specificity, thus indicating that the immune system is extremely flexible.

2. Antibodies to structurally complex haptens exhibit specificity for only a portion of the total hapten molecule, reflecting a limitation on the size of the antibody-combining site.

3. Haptenic structure is an important limiting factor in the affinity of antihapten antibodies. The highest-affinity antibodies are obtained to large, structurally complex, hydrophobic haptens.

4. The antibody-hapten interaction involves a summation of binding energies, including hydrophobic, charge-transfer, hydrogen-bonding, and Coulombic forces. The pattern is determined by the structure of the hapten, helping explain why different antibody-hapten systems differ markedly in how they are affected by changes in ionic strength, pH, and temperature. Charged haptens, for example, interact with oppositely charged amino

acid residues in the antibody-combining region, and binding is likely to be sensitive both to variations in pH and to ionic strength.

5. The antibody responses to proteins may be directed toward sequential, conformational, or haptenic determinants. Much or all of the response is directed toward sterically accessible areas on the native protein rather than determinants unmasked as the protein is degraded.

6. The magnitude and specificity of the anti-protein response are influenced by the genetic makeup of the animal and by how foreign the protein is. As a rule, a number of structurally distinct areas on the protein stimulate antibody formation. A number of these determinants can be occupied simultaneously by antibody. In other words, most proteins contain a number of independent antigenic domains, each producing and interacting with its own particular antibody.

7. Immunological cross-reactivity occurs between proteins that have areas of homology in portions of their amino acid sequences.

8. In general, when a protein undergoes polymerization, part of its antigenic determinants are masked. Less frequently, new specificities appear. When a protein undergoes degradation, new antigenic determinants almost certainly will be created. Preexisting antigenic determinants may or may not be destroyed.

9. It is sometimes possible to use chemical or enzymatic degradation techniques and obtain protein fragments containing isolated antigenic determinants. This is a useful approach to problems of immunological cross-reactivity.

10. The specificity of antiprotein antibodies may change during the course of immunization, probably reflecting competition between different antigenic determinants on the same protein molecule.

11. Under favorable circumstances antibodies can distinguish between two very closely related proteins that differ by as little as one amino acid residue.

Chapter 5

Indicator Molecules

INTRODUCTION

The indicator molecule may be attached either to antigen or antibody and radioactivity, enzymatic activity, electron spin resonance, or fluorescence used as a marker. Until now, radioactive molecules have been the most sensitive and flexible markers, but this situation may change as further theoretical and technical developments occur.

RADIOACTIVE MARKERS

General Considerations

There are a number of approaches to the introduction of a radioactive label. A radioactive precurser can be incorporated into the primary structure of an antigen during organic or biological synthesis, resulting in a molecule that is essentially unaltered structurally (intrinsic labeling). Alternatively, chemical or enzymatic techniques can be used to introduce label into already completed molecules of antigen (terminal labeling). In terminal labeling procedures the label can be introduced directly, provided that the antigen contains amino acid or other residues that are easily and stably labeled. Where a suitable target for labeling is not available, it is often possible to introduce a susceptible residue chemically prior to labeling. Another approach involves the incorporation of the radioactive marker into an immunologically unrelated carrier molecule that is secondarily attached to antigen. Or if a metal or some other cofactor is tightly bound to the antigen, labeling by exchange with a radioactive ligand may be possible. The selection of a radiolabeling procedure is determined by the sensitivity requirements and structural characteristics of the immune system in question. They include

1. The quantity of unlabeled antigen that must be measured.
2. The susceptibility of the antigen to chemical or physical denatura-

tion during or after labeling and the influence this factor will have on specific and nonspecific binding.

3. The availability of the purified antigen or antigen derivative that is used for labeling.

4. The ease and reproducibility of labeling.

5. The convenience of processing large numbers of immunoassay samples for separation of bound and unbound antigen and counting.

6. The stability of radiolabeled antigen under standard immunoassay conditions in the presence of serum or tissue components.

A new immunoassay system presents special problems that must be worked out empirically, but, as a rule, reasonable predictions as to an optimal method of labeling are possible.

Choosing an Isotope

A critical factor in the choice of a radioactive marker is the specific activity of the isotope. The half lives of ^{131}I (8 days), ^{125}I (60 days), ^{14}C (5,730 years), and ^{3}H (12.3 years) (Catch, 1971) differ greatly. The importance of half life in radioactive emission is evident when the relative specific activities of the different isotopes are calculated. Specific activities are expressed in millicuries (mCi) or curies (Ci). By definition, one millicurie represents 2.2×10^{9} radioactive disintegrations/minute and one curie is one thousandfold higher; atoms of ^{131}I, ^{125}I, ^{3}H, and ^{14}C have specific activities of 19,250, 2,560, 33, and 0.07 Ci/mmole, respectively. The introduction of a single atom of ^{131}I into a molecule of bovine insulin provides about 1,000 times the number of radioactive disintegrations per unit time as would be obtained if all 263 carbon atoms in the molecule were labeled with ^{14}C (Hunter, 1967). And 586 atoms of ^{3}H give off the same number of radioactive disintegrations per unit time as one molecule of ^{131}I (Hunter, 1967). Depending on the radioactive counter used, the advantage of ^{131}I over ^{3}H may be further increased; ^{131}I can be counted with about 40 to 80% efficiency, whereas ^{3}H is counted with an efficiency that varies between 15 and 40%.

With a radioactive marker of low specific activity, relatively high concentrations of marker are required in order to obtain a practical level of radioactivity in the immunoassay. For example, if the specific activity of a ^{3}H-labeled hapten is 1 mCi/mmole, in order to obtain a total of 5,000 counts per minute (cpm) (about the minimal number of counts that might be used in a radioimmunoassay if unduly long counting times are to be avoided), 5.7 nmoles of marker would be needed (assuming 40% counting efficiency). When the quantity of radiolabeled hapten used in the assay is this large, substantial amounts of antibody must be used to maintain labeled hapten binding at the desired level (at least 20 to 30% binding, see below), Regardless of the affinity of the antibody, this immunoassay system would be relatively insensitive. As a rough rule of thumb, when the quantity of unlabeled hapten in a competitive immunoassay is much below 25% of the labeled hapten present, changes in marker binding will be difficult to detect. When the addition of labeled antigen is delayed until after the antibody has equilibrated with unlabeled antigen, it may be possible to detect amounts of unlabeled antigen that are as low as 5% of the total radiolabeled antigen present. Of course, if the unlabeled hapten is recognized more readily than the marker by the antibody, more favorable ratios might be obtained.

The use of a radioiodinated marker has additional important advantages. ^{125}I and ^{131}I can be counted in ordinary test tubes in well-type gamma counters, and transfer before counting is not necessary. ^{3}H and ^{14}C must be counted by liquid scintillation, which requires the use of expensive scintillation solutions and counting vials, plus the expenditure of extra time in processing samples. Moreover, when an attempt is made to increase marker specific activity by maximizing the number of radioactive atoms of ^{3}H or ^{14}C incorporated per molecule, rapid decomposition sometimes occurs (Evans, 1966), resulting in a practical level of radioactivity that is considerably below the theoretical maximum. This is also a problem with heavily radioiodinated products; but at comparable levels of radioactivity, an antigen that is lightly substituted with iodine may fare much better than an antigen that is heavily substituted with ^{3}H or ^{14}C.

With many proteins, loss of antigenic reactivity is as much a function of the absolute number of iodine atoms incorporated as it is of specific activity per se. Where a marker of high specific activity is needed, it might be assumed that ^{131}I, with a half life of 8 days, would have a marked advantage over ^{125}I, with a half life of 60 days, but such is not the case.

1. Commercially available preparations of "carrier-free" ^{131}I contain up 80 to 85% ^{127}I, whereas the degree of contamination of ^{125}I is much less, probably less than 4% (Freedlender, 1969; Greenwood, 1971). Thus in order to obtain comparable labeling of protein, the total number of iodine atoms that must be introduced is comparable with ^{125}I and ^{131}I (or, at best, only about 40% fewer iodine atoms with fresh ^{131}I).

2. Any possible advantage ^{131}I might have is nullified completely by the relatively low counting efficiency of some commercially available gamma counters for ^{131}I (40 to 80%, as compared with 80% for ^{125}I) (Hunter, 1967).

3. The short life of ^{131}I is a disadvantage in that the shelf life of antigens labeled with this isotope is limited. Any preparation of ^{131}I-or ^{131}I-labeled protein that is more than 8 days old has lost at least 50% of its original radioactivity. ^{125}I-labeled antigens can be used for several weeks with relatively little fall in specific activity.

4. Compounds containing ^{125}I tend to be more stable than those with ^{131}I because of the absence of Beta radiation (Catch, 1971).

5. The gamma radiation given off by ^{125}I is less energetic than that of ^{131}I and penetrates much less readily through glass and clothing. [125]I is therefore less of a radiation hazard than ^{131}I for laboratory personnel. This factor is significant in laboratories doing extensive immunoassay work, particularly those carrying out their own iodination reactions.

Thus considering the differences in isotope abundance, counting efficiency, half life, stability, and external radiation hazard, ^{125}I is normally preferred to [131]I.

Direct Radioiodination of Protein Antigens

IODINATION WITH CHLORAMINE T

A variety of possible chemical methods for introducing iodine onto proteins exist (Ramachandran, 1956). The most widely used radioiodination procedure for proteins involves the use of chloramine T, the N-chloro-derivative of p-methylbenzenesulfonamide, a mild oxidizing agent. The reagent has been in widespread use since 1962, when Hunter and Greenwood (1962) showed that low concentrations of chloramine T promoted highly efficient incorporation of inorganic iodide into protein. The chloramine T procedure was an improvement over earlier methods of iodinating proteins in terms of rapidity and reproducibility, the avoidance of organic solvents or extremes of pH that might denature protein, and an ability to obtain efficient iodination in the absence of carrier, nonradioactive iodide. The mechanism of the reaction has not been carefully studied, but it is probable that it involves the generation of cationic [I^+] iodine, which is a potent oxidizing agent. Introduction of radioactive iodine atoms onto the protein occurs through an electrophilic substitution of the charged phenolic hydroxyl group on tyrosyl residues. As discussed below, substitution of iodine onto histidyl imidazole, or cysteinyl sulfhydryl groups is also possible.

A representative protocol for chloramine T iodination is given in Table 5.1. In the example shown, the quantity of protein ($20\mu g$) and ^{125}I radioactivity (1 mCi) was selected to provide a product of high specific activity.

Reactions are carried out in a small (30 to 200 μliters) volume, which permits the iodination of minute amounts of protein at sufficiently high protein concentrations to achieve an efficient utilization of radioiodine. Iodination efficiency is markedly affected by protein concentration. For

Table 5.1

Chloramine T Iodination.

1. ^{125}I, 1 mCi	0.01 ml
2. Phosphate buffer, 0.5 M, pH 7.6	0.10 ml
3. Protein (HGH), 20 μg	0.02 ml
4. Chloramine T, 180 μg *	0.05 ml
5. Stir 20–30 seconds at room temperature	
6. Na metabisulfite, 500 μg *	0.05 ml
7. Immediately apply to Sephadex G-50 column packed in 0.15 M NaCl–0.01 M PO_4 (PBS)	
8. Collect and pool initial radioactivity peak (iodinated protein) (see Fig. 5.4)	
9. Dilute in PBS containing 10 mg/ml bovine serum albumin	
10. Store at 4°C (short-term use) or frozen	

A representative procedure for protein iodinated by the chloramine T method. (Taken from Peake, 1974.)

* The chloramine T and sodium metabisulfite solutions are prepared immediately before use in 0.01 M phosphate buffer. Note that absolute amounts of protein, ^{125}I, chloramine T, and metabisulfite are given in the table, rather than concentrations. As part of the column preparation, the column had been primed with a 1-ml bolus of a 1 to 5 mg/ml solution of bovine serum albumin in PBS. The procedure can easily be scaled down or up by proportionate reductions or increases in the volumes of the reactants.

proteins with a moderate tyrosine content, incorporation of iodine falls from 100% at 1 mg of protein/ml to 60 to 70% at 50 μg of protein/ml (Hunter, 1973). In order to obtain high levels of radioactivity while keeping the reaction volume to a minimum, concentrated solutions of radioiodine (100 mCi/ml or higher) are used, thus permitting the addition of 1 mCi or more in a volume of only 10 μliters. Concentrated solutions of ^{125}I contain significant concentrations of NaOH (up to 0.1 M), and the protein should be well buffered before the radioiodine is added. The use of 0.2 to 0.5 M phosphate, pH 7.2 to 8.4 (or borate, in the same pH range), provides adequate buffering capacity while bringing the pH into a range that is appropriate for iodination. The optimal pH for iodination varies, but for most proteins a pH between 7.3 and 7.8 provides effective labeling (Fig. 5.1). Some investigators avoid having chloride ion in the

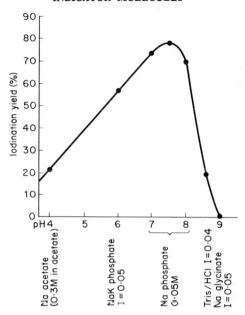

Fig. 5.1. Effect of pH on the efficiency of iodination. Human-growth hormone (HGH) (100 μg) was reacted with iodide (40 ng) as Na ^{127}I plus a trace amount of Na ^{131}I. (Taken from W. M. Hunter. 1973. *In* D. M. Weir (Ed.). Handbook of experimental immunology. Blackwell Scientific Publications, Oxford. pp. 17.1–17.36.)

reaction mixture, chloride being a halide ion and susceptible to oxidation. However, the oxidation of I⁻ is so much more efficient that Cl⁻ that satisfactory iodination can be obtained, even at Cl⁻ concentrations of 0.1 *M* or higher.

Oxidation of iodine takes place rapidly after the introduction of chloramine T into the iodination mixture, and rapid mixing is needed to prevent uneven labelings. The reaction is allowed to proceed for anywhere from a few seconds to 10 minutes at 0 to 24°C (usually one minute or less). An excess of sodium metabisulfite, a reducing agent, is then added to stop the reaction. A 1.2 to 1.5-fold molar excess of metabisulfite over chloramine T is sufficient to reduce all the unreacted chloramine T. Once the chloramine T has been reduced, carrier-heterologous protein can be added directly to the iodination mixture. The quantity of chloramine T must be adequate to neutralize the small amount of reducing agent normally present in the Na^{125}I and allow for possible side reactions with protein, as well as oxidize the I⁻. The chloramine T dose dependency for iodination of bovine albumin is shown in Fig. 5.2. Somewhat surprisingly, it takes more chloramine T during iodination with carrier-free ^{125}I than with equivalent quan-

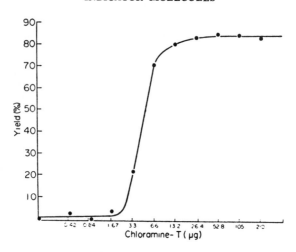

Fig. 5.2. Chloramine-T requirement for iodination. 100 μg of BSA was reacted with 100 ng [127]I (as KI) plus a trace amount of Na [131]I. Note the inefficient iodination at low chloramine T concentrations. (Taken from W. M. Hunter. 1973. *In* D. M. Weir (Ed.). Handbook of experimental immunology. Blackwell Scientific Publications, Oxford. pp. 17.1–17.36.)

tities of [127]I (Hunter, 1974). The level of protein iodination is affected by the concentration and duration of exposure to chloramine T. Both are kept to a minimum so as to avoid nonspecific chloramine T damage to the protein (Yalow and Berson, 1971). Optimal reaction conditions should be determined for each protein, depending on the desired specific activity, tyrosine reactivity, and protein susceptibility to iodination or chloramine T damage (see below). When dealing with a new protein antigen, it may be desirable to begin by tagging it lightly with [125]I (approximately one iodine atom per 10 or 20 protein molecules) so as to minimize the possibility of reduction in immunologic reactivity during labeling (Hunter, 1974). The labeled protein can then be used as an indicator molecule to detect losses in antigenic reactivity in other preparations of antigen that are exposed to more severe iodination conditions. Additional antigen is reacted with various quantities of [127]I and chloramine T or chloramine T alone for several time periods and evaluated as an inhibitor of radioactive antigen binding by antibody (Fig. 5.3). If there are marked losses of inhibitory activity as compared with the native (unlabeled and unreacted) antigen, an unacceptable loss of antigenic reactivity has probably occurred.

As a rule, the goal will be to substitute an average of about one atom of I per molecule of antigen. A molecule of protein that contains less than one atom of iodine is not labeled at all, and ordinarily little is gained by having most of the protein molecules unlabeled. The substitution of multiple atoms of iodine will often result in substantial losses of antigenic reactivity,

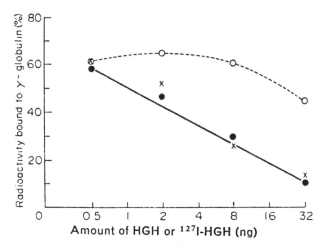

Fig. 5.3. Comparison of [127]I-HGH and unlabeled HGH in regard to their ability to compete with a small amount of ^{131}I-HGH for antibody-binding sites. The [127]I-HGH contained: •, 0.7 atom [127]I/molecule; X, 7 atoms of [127]I/molecule; o, 14 atoms of [127]I/molecule. The solid line represents unlabeled HGH (experimental points omitted). (Taken from F. C. Greenwood, W. M. Hunter, and J. S. Glover. 1963. Biochem. J. 89:114–123.)

as discussed in detail below. Where this is true, the gain in specific activity will be more than counterbalanced by the unfavorable change in antigen binding.

Purification is carried out immediately after iodination in order to remove unconjugated iodine oxidation products, free iodide and reducing agent. The separation can be accomplished by various methods. In general, the reaction mixture is chromatographed on a molecular sieve, such as Sephadex G-25 or G-50 (Fig. 5.4) (Peake, 1974). The gel is primed with a heterologous, non-cross-reacting protein, such as bovine serum albumin or ovalbumin, in order to reduce nonspecific absorption of the radiolabeled protein. If marked damage to antigen occurs during iodination, it may be desirable to try to separate the damaged from the undamaged antigen as part of the initial purification procedure. Depending on the protein, this process may be done by electrophoresis on starch or polyacrylamide gel or by chromatography on an ion exchange or affinity column.

IODINATION WITH LACTOPEROXIDASE

An interesting approach to protein (or hapten) iodination involves the use of the oxidizing enzyme, lactoperoxidase, a 90,000-molecular-weight protein obtained from unpasteurized bovine milk (Marchalonis 1969; Morrison et al., 1971). In the presence of low concentrations of hydrogen

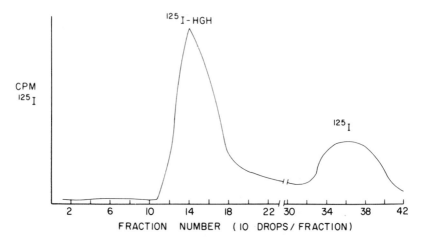

Fig. 5.4. Elution pattern of ^{125}I from Sephadex G-50 following the iodination of human-growth hormone. (Taken from G. T. Peake. 1974. In B. M. Jaffe, and H. R. Behrman (Eds.). Methods of hormone radioimmunoassay. Academic Press, New York. pp. 103–123.)

peroxide, the enzyme will iodinate soluble and insoluble proteins. The iodination is principally on tyrosyl residues, although histidyl and sulhydryl groups may also participate. The reaction is enzymatic in nature and has been shown to involve three substrates—peroxide, iodide, and the phenolic compound that is being iodinated (Morrison et al., 1971). The efficiency of iodination is determined by the absolute concentrations of the target protein, the enzyme, hydrogen peroxide, and iodide (Figs. 5.5 and 5.6).

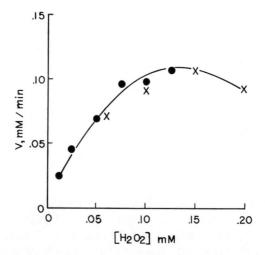

Fig. 5.5. H_2O_2 optimum at pH 7.4 for lactoperoxidase iodination of tyrosine. (●———●) mono-iodotyrosine production, (X———X) I^- disappearance. (Taken from M. Morrison, and G. S. Bayse. 1970. Biochemistry. 9:2995–3000.)

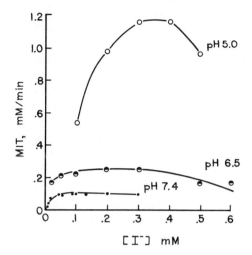

Fig. 5.6. Effect of iodide concentration on rate of iodination of L-tyrosine by lactoperoxidase at optimal concentrations of H_2O_2 and tyrosine. (Taken from M. Morrison, and G. S. Bayse. 1970. Biochemistry. 9:2995–3000.)

A representative iodination using lactoperoxidase is shown in Table 5.2. In general, relatively crude commercial preparations of lactoperoxidase are satisfactory, although their use does increase the quantity of contaminating protein in the reaction mixture (see below). The H_2O_2 can be added as such or generated in the iodination solution by the reaction of glucose oxidase with D-glucose. High concentrations of H_2O_2 (>100 μM) inhibit

Table 5.2

Lactoperoxidase Iodination.

1. 1.8 mCi ^{125}I	0.015 ml
2. Protein (bovine insulin) 5 μg in 0.05 PO_4, pH 7.5	0.025 ml
3. Lactoperoxidase, 4 μg in above buffer * †	0.0015 ml
4. H_2O_2, 0.88 mmole †	0.001 ml
5. Stir 60 seconds at room temperature	
6. 0.05 M phosphate, pH 7.4	0.500 ml
7. Immediately apply to 20 ml Sephadex G-25 column, packed in PBS, and process as in Table 5.1.	

A representative procedure for protein iodination by the lactoperoxidase method. The procedure given is for purified lactoperoxidase with an A_{412} nmole/A_{280} nmole ratio of 0.8 to 0.9. However, similar levels of iodination can be obtained with larger amounts of less pure lactoperoxidase. According to the authors, 96% of the 1.8 mCi of ^{125}I was incorporated into insulin by this method. (Taken from Thorell and Johansson, 1971.)

* Procedures using much smaller concentrations of lactoperoxidase (2.4 $\mu g/ml$) have also been described (see, for example, Morrison, Bayse, and Webster, 1971).

† The H_2O_2 and lactoperoxidase are diluted shortly before use.

the enzyme (Fig. 5.5), but since the concentrations of H_2O_2 used for iodination (1 to 20 μM) are much lower, enzyme inactivation is not a problem. As a rule, the quantity of H_2O_2 added can be used to control the level of iodination, with close to one mole of iodine being incorporated per mole of H_2O_2. However, some preparations of radioiodine contain small amount of H_2O_2, thus resulting in higher levels of iodination than had been calculated. The rate of reaction with tyrosine and most proteins is maximal at pH 4.5 to 5.0 (Morrison et al., 1971) (Fig. 5.5), but with certain proteins the optimal may be nearer neutrality. In general, relatively efficient iodination is obtained over a pH range from 3.0 to 8.0, which permits the selection of a pH that gives optimal selectivity of labeling, depending on the protein or peptide. Under optimal conditions the introduction of iodine into proteins is rapid, even exceeding the rate of iodination with chloramine T. Lactoperoxidase has been shown to catalyse the incorporation into bovine albumin of up to 6.5 $\times$ 10^3 moles of iodine/mole protein/minute (at pH 7.4) (Morrison et al., 1971). The rate of reaction with free tyrosine is more than an order of magnitude faster (Morrison and Bayse, 1974). The K_m for iodide and free tyrosine varies with the reaction conditions with representative values of 5 and 50 mmole, respectively (Morrison and Bayse, 1974). The reaction can be stopped or markedly retarded by adding 10 or 20 volumes of cold buffer, followed by chromatographic fractionation. If instantaneous inhibition is required, a reducing agent, such as cysteine, can be included in the diluent. Insolubilized preparations of lactoperoxidase (coupled to Sepharose by the cyanogen bromide reaction) can be used in order to facilitate the removal of the enzyme after the iodination reaction is completed (David, 1972). Or the iodinated proteins can be separated from lactoperoxidase and unconjugated iodine by a suitable chromatographic procedure. Physical removal of the lactoperoxidase either by centrifugation or by chromatography may be desirable because lactoperoxidase itself can be iodinated—in effect, introducing an iodinated protein contaminant into the antigen (Thorell and Johansson, 1971). Normally, however, the target protein is labeled so much faster than lactoperoxidase, even at high lactoperoxidase concentrations, that self-iodination of lactoperoxidase is not a problem. With an antigen that labels inefficiently, a high antigen concentration, together with a one hundredfold lower concentration of lactoperoxidase, may help to minimize the iodination of the enzyme.

Problems in lactoperoxidase iodination can arise from the use of too high a concentration of H_2O_2 or from the use of partially inactivated H_2O_2 or lactoperoxidase. H_2O_2 is unstable in dilute solution and is therefore stored as a concentrated 30% solution at 4°C and diluted just before use. Since catalases are widely distributed in tissue and react rapidly with H_2O_2, the possibility that trace amounts are present in the incubation mixture and are competing with lactoperoxidase may need to be considered. On the other hand, as discussed above, when large amounts of radioactive iodine are used, the reaction, may proceed spontaneously in the absence of exogenous H_2O_2 because of small amounts of H_2O_2 in the radioactive iodine (Thorell and Johansson, 1971). Ideally, the lactoperoxidase should be freshly dissolved and diluted, although if concentrated solutions of the enzyme are stored under optimal conditions, most of the iodination activity is preserved for at least several days. There are also potential problems due to variation in commercial lots of lactoperoxidase or changes in activity of the lyophillized protein with age, and it may be desirable to determine the activity of the lactoperoxidase directly. A modification of the fluorometric assay procedure of Keston and Brandt (1965) may be used for this purpose, although a direct measurement of protein-iodinating activity under conditions in which lactoperoxidase is limiting should be equally satisfactory. The fluorometric procedure involves the oxidation of dichlorofluorescin (nonfluorescent) to dichlorofluorescein (fluorescent) in the presence of H_2O_2 and a peroxidase. It was described originally as a means of measuring H_2O_2 by using horseradish peroxidase as the oxidizing enzyme, but it is readily adapted to the measurement of either horseradish peroxidase or lactoperoxidase (C. W. Parker, unpublished observations). Problems can also occur if the enzyme is contaminated with proteases or if the antigen solution contains one of the reducing agents that interferes with lactoperoxidase activtiy. Azide, for example, is frequently used as a preservative for protein and is a potent inhibitor of lactoperoxidase (Thorell and Johansson, 1971). For reasons that are not entirely clear, difficulties also seem to occur in catalytic iodination with certain lots of radioactive iodine.

The ease with which soluble proteins are iodinated with lactoperoxidase varies considerably with the protein, reflecting, in large measure, the extent of association between the enzyme and the protein. Enzymatic iodination is a less random process than chemical iodination and is favored in regions of the target protein that contain tyrosyl residues that are sterically available to the enzyme. The directed nature of enzymatic iodination is illustrated by a study with bovine insulin that used horseradish peroxidase rather than lactoperoxidase as the iodinating enzyme (see below). By a proper choice of enzymatic iodination conditions, it was possible to obtain preparations in which 90% of the ^{125}I was on the tyrosine at the 19 position of the A chain (Lambert and Jacquemin, 1973). When chemical iodination methods are used, the label is equally distributed between the A_{14} and $_{19}$ tyrosines. Similar results have been obtained with lactoperoxidase and ferricytochrome C, where enzymatic labeling leads to substitution of exposed tyrosyls only (at position 74) but chemical iodination involves buried tyrosyls as well (Morrison and Bayse, 1974). In addition to selecting for accessible tyrosyls, use of a peroxidase also markedly increases the probability of obtaining monoiodo rather than diiodotyrosyl on the protein.

Thus enzymatically labeled proteins will usually be more homogeneous than chemically iodinated proteins. The selectivity of lactoperoxidase iodination may be an important advantage with proteins that are unusually subject to damage during chloramine T iodination. Enzymatic iodination may also be useful in the iodination of histidyl residues (in hormones, such as secretin, which do not contain phenolic hydroxyl groups) (Holohan et al., 1973). The N-terminal histidine of secretin has been labeled by using this method, iodination occurring at a pH optimum of 6.0. Iodination of imidazole groups does not occur readily in the chloramine T method, for high levels of alkalinity and oxidant are generally required.

Other peroxidases are capable of catalysing protein iodination, including horseradish peroxidase, thyroid peroxidase, chloroperoxidase, and myeloperoxidase. These enzymes have a lower iodination efficiency for proteins than lactoperoxidase. This fact is particularly true of horseradish peroxidase, which has a specific activity for protein that is more than three orders of magnitude below that of lactoperoxidase (Morrison and Bayse, 1974). Whether it will be advantageous to evaluate other peroxidases when lactoperoxidase does not give satisfactory labeling is not yet clear. Horseradish peroxidase (40,000, M.W.) is considerably smaller than lactoperoxidase (90,000, M.W.), thus possibly increasing the area on the protein surface with which it might establish effective contact and altering the selectivity of the reaction.

The extent to which the lactoperoxidase method will supplant the chloramine T method for routine iodination purposes is uncertain. Thorell and Johansson (1971) have studied the immunoassay performance of proteins iodinated by the lactoperoxidase method, choosing a group of commonly measured hormones (glucagon, growth hormone, insulin, LH, TSH, and FSH) for analysis. They obtained labeled antigens that were highly immunoreactive, exhibiting more than 80% binding in the presence of excess antibody with very little evidence of denaturation. Morrison et al. (1971) were able to incorporate up to 12 atoms of iodine into bovine serum albumin with little or no change in its antigenic reactivity. Miyachi and Chrambach (1972) analyzed FSH, HCG, and LH by polyacrylamide gel electrophoresis after chloramine T and lactoperoxidase iodination and observed that gross changes in net charge and protein conformation occurred only in chloramine T- oxidized preparations. Taken together, these findings suggest that the lactoperoxidase method will ultimately find widespread application. Certainly, for proteins subject to oxidation damage, enzymatic iodination should be highly advantageous (see below).

OTHER IODINATION TECHNIQUES

Iodine monochloride. Another useful method for iodination utilizes iodine monochloride (ICl) as the reactant (McFarlane, 1965). Radiolabeled ^{125}I is first oxidized to$^{125}I_2$, which is then equilibrated with ^{127}ICl and reacted with protein (Ceska et al., 1971).

Historically, the use of ICl for protein iodination came before chloramine T but has been largely superseded (Odell et a. 1967). The major disadvantage of the iodine monochloride method is the necessity for carrier ^{125}I, which decreases iodination efficiency and lowers the specific activity of the product (Ceska et al., 1971). However, with selected proteins, the ICl method produces considerably less protein denaturation than chloramine T. Therefore the ICl method may warrant evaluation in the event that chloramine T oxidation experiments have given disappointing results.

Electrolytic iodination. Another method that is said to minimize damage to protein is iodination in an electrolytic cell. A solution of the protein I⁻ at neutral pH is placed in an electric field. Elementary iodine is released at the anode and reacts with the protein (Rosa et al., 1967). Unfortunately, this method is not easily adaptable to iodination in small volumes.

Oxidation of iodide by chlorine gas. Still another procedure involves the ability of gaseous chlorine to convert radioactive iodide to iodine (Butt, 1972; Hunter, 1974).

Special Problems Associated with Iodination

Problems associated with the radioiodination of proteins include radiolabeling of trace impurities, losses of antigen reactivity occurring during iodination, or decomposition on storage (Catch, 1971).

IODINATION OF IMPURITIES

Iodination of impure antigens may pose special problems if a contaminating protein is more readily iodinated than the antigen itself. In this case, a trace contaminant may contain most of the radioactivity, thus resulting in preparations that are not optimal for immunoassay studies. This problem arose in early chloramine T experiments with hepatitis B antigen, where in preparations of antigen that appeared more than 95% pure chromatographically, over 80% of the radioactivity was incorporated into proteinaceous impurities (Aach and Parker, unpublished data). If the contaminating protein, free of the antigen, is available in quantity, the specificity of binding may be improved by absorbing the antibody with the contaminant or by performing the assay routinely in the presence of excess unlabeled contaminating protein. Carefully chosen iodination conditions may provide better selectivity, with a greater degree of labeling of antigen and a lesser degree of labeling of the contaminant. Finally, more rigorous purification of the antigen may be needed. Depending on the protein, this process may be better accomplished before or after iodination.

A special problem may arise with complex antigens like lipoproteins, mammalian cells, or viruses, where radioiodine may form unstable complexes with lipids or other constituents in addition to stable complexes with proteins. In this case, the iodinated particle may release iodine slowly and so complicate the interpretation of immunological studies. The use of lactoperoxidase should largely circumvent this problem. Morrison and his colleagues (1971) have observed that when influenza-X7 virus is iodinated by the lactoperoxidase reaction, only 0.2% of the total iodine incorporated is in the lipid fraction, whereas, with chemical iodination, extensive iodination of viral lipid occurs.

ANTIGENIC ALTERATIONS

The kinds of antigenic alteration possible during iodination vary widely, reflecting (a) the introduction of iodine per se, (b) side reactions involving noniodinatable but oxidizable amino acid residues, (c) denaturation associated with dilution and manipulation of the purified protein, and (d) problems associated with impurities in the radioactive iodine.

Changes associated with the introduction of iodine. The most prominent protein modification produced by oxidative iodination is formation of mono- and diiodotyrosyl groups. The reaction of I_2 or I^+ with tyrosyl appears to involve the negative-charged phenolate group and thus explains the greater efficiency of iodination in neutral or weakly alkaline solutions (Mayberry et al., 1965). Iodination of tyrosine is less efficient in more strongly alkaline solutions, probably because of more rapid hydrolysis of oxidized iodine and the occurrence of side reactions with other functional groups on the protein (such as histidyl). Diiodination is ordinarily favored, presumably because the lower pK_a of monoiodophenol favors the introduction of a second I atom once monoiodination has occurred. Much of the monoiodotyrosine found following the hydrolysis of iodinated proteins appears to be an artifact of the hydrolysis itself (Hunter, 1967). Lactoperoxidase iodination is an exception in that monoiodination of tyrosine is the favored reaction (Lambert and Jacquemin, 1973).

In addition to tyrosine, uptake of iodine is also possible on histidyl and sulfhydryl groups. As noted, during iodination with chloramine T, histidine residues generally are not attacked unless an unusually high pH and chloramine T concentration is used. It is possible, however, that a histidyl residue might be unusually reactive to I^+, analogous to the well-recognized high reactivity of the two histidyl residues in the active site of alkylating agents or the high reactivity of serine hydroxyl groups in the active center of serine esterases. Unwanted histidyl iodination is more likely to be a problem with lactoperoxidase, which is capable of introducing iodine onto histidine under relatively mild conidtions, although if tyrosyl residues are also present, they would be expected to react preferentially. Morrison and Bayse (1974) have shown that although histidine and tyrosine compete for the same binding site on lactoperoxidase, the K_m is more than twentyfold higher for histidine than for tyrosine. Sulfhydryl groups may react with oxidized iodine to form sulfenyl iodides and sulfenyl periodides, some of which are unstable and break down to regenerate SH or form uncharacterized products (Jirousek and Pritchard, 1971).

Iodination of critical tyrosines. Although the total number of iodine molecules that can be introduced onto a protein or polypeptide is determined largely by its overall tyrosine content, the likelihood that damage will occur under ordinary labeling conditions is more a reflection of individual tyrosine distribution and reactivity. If a major antigenic group on a protein contains a tyrosyl residue and the tyrosyl is labeled with iodine, loss of antigenic reactivity will probably occur. The likelihood that a critical tyrosine will be labeled will increase as the level of protein iodination is increased, which explains in part why high levels of iodination are more likely to be associated with unacceptable losses of antigenic reactivity than lower levels of labeling.

In considering the problem of direct iodination damage, it is useful to determine the number of iodine atoms being introduced onto the protein. The conversion from counts per minute per milligram iodinated protein to atoms of iodine-introduced protein molecule is easily made, provided that the protein molecular weight, counting efficiency, and isotope abundance are known.

As discussed earlier, in commercially available radioactive iodines, the relative isotope abundance of ^{125}I is in excess of 95%, whereas the figure for ^{131}I is about 25%. A useful figure to keep in mind is that fresh preparations of ^{125}I contain 4×10^{-7} mmoles of iodide/mCi.

The number of tyrosyl residues per molecule in a number of commonly iodinated antigens and the specific activities obtained in practical immunoassays are given in Table 5.3. For most hormones, a specific activity of 100 to 500 $\mu Ci/\mu g$ protein is readily obtained without substantial losses of immunologic reactivity.

Nonspecific effects of heavy iodination. As already indicated, in addition to inactivation due to the substitution of critical tyrosines, heavy iodine substitution per se may be detrimental. Attempts to utilize protein antigens that are very heavily labeled with radioiodine for radioimmunoassays are often unsuccessful because of decreases in specific binding activity and an increased tendency of the protein to aggregate and bind nonspecifically. Heavily iodinated proteins contain large amounts of diiodotyrosine, and diiodotyrosine is in the form of the negatively charged diiophenolate ion at neutral pH. Thus as the level of iodination increases, the protein be-

Table 5.3

Theoretical and actual specific activities for some iodinated-polypeptide-hormone antigens used in sensitive hormone immuno-assay measurements.

| Hormone | Molecular weight | Tyrosyls/ molecule | ^{125}I Specific activity mCi/ml | | |
			For 1 radio-active atom/ molecule	For fully iodinated molecule	Specific activity in representative preparations used for immunoassay
Glucagon	~3,500	2	~650	~2,600	~300–500
ACTH	~4,500	2	~510	~2,040	~100–400
Insulin	~6,000	4	~380	~3,040	~150–220
Parathyroid (beef)	~9,000	1	~250	~500	~200–400
HGH	~2,000	0	~115	~1,040	~30–100

Theoretical calculations are made using 18 mCi/μg as the specific activity of carrier-free ^{125}I. The specific activities of representative immunoassay-iodinated antigen preparations are taken from Odell and Daughaday (1971), Jaffe and Behrman (1974), or individual papers. Modified from Yalow and Berson (Table II, 1969).

comes more anionic. The change in charge is sufficient to permit the separation of different iodinated species of a single protein on an anion exchange resin and may be a factor in the reduction in antigenic reactivity seen in extensively iodinated proteins. However, changes in tertiary structure and increased aggregation are probably more important. Increased aggregation is especially likely to occur with chloramine T, having been noted with intact and fragmented human fibrinogen, human albumin, human IgG, human LH, and bovine and ovine growth hormone (Sherman et al., 1974). Chloramine T alone produces these changes, indicating that reactive free radicals produced by radiation are not involved. Apparently this complication is much less likely to occur with ICl iodination, and for this reason investigators who are interested in studying the biological half life of labeled proteins in vivo often prefer the ICl method.

Oxidation damage. Oxidation is another factor in altered protein re-activity, and it, too, will vary markedly with the protein. Disulfide, indole, and thioether groups may be altered during iodination without the intro-duction of iodine molecules per se. Alterations of this kind are sometimes associated with adverse effects on antigenic reactivity, although this is by no means always the case. Fortunately, chloramine T can be used under relatively mild conditions so that most proteins escape or are little altered by oxidation. The damage may be produced by the oxidizing agent itself or by oxidized iodine. The different iodination procedures vary in their tendency to produce oxidation damage, although some degree of damage is at least theoretically possible with all of them. Lactoperoxidase iodination involves the lowest risk of adventitious oxidation. While it is true that the protein is exposed to low levels of H_2O_2, during enzymatic iodination the level of free H_2O_2 need not exceed 10×10^{-6} M, which is unlikely to result in damage. The oxidized forms of iodine themselves are not free in the medium but are transferred directly to tyrosine, thus reducing the exposure of the protein as a whole to oxidation.

The nature of the oxidative damage produced during labeling varies with the protein. Chloramine T-induced changes have been the most extensively studied. Damage due to chloramine T oxidation is more likely to occur during unusually rigorous iodination conditions, but with susceptible proteins even a brief exposure to low concentrations of reagent may be harmful. The oxidation may involve disulfide bonds or methionyl or tryptophanyl residues. Oxidation of disulfide bonds is a complication of chloramine T iodination of insulin, whereas methionine oxidation presents problems when parathormone (Repke and Zull, 1972; Zull and Repke, 1972) or flagellin (Parish and Stanley, 1972) is labeled. The methionine residues of flagellin are also oxidized with changes occurring at the 111 and 331 positions of the molecule (Parish and Stanley, 1972). However, even a complete conversion of the two methionines does not adversely affect the antigenicity or immunogenicity of the protein despite an alteration of its polymerizing properties.

Alexander (1974) has studied the effect of iodination on free tryptophan and tryptophanyl-containing peptides. Tryptophanyl groups were oxidized by chloramine T, N-iodosuccinmide, lactoperoxidase, and horseradish peroxidase. The reaction rate was maximal at or near pH 5 but extended into the alkaline range. The oxidation was accompanied by cleavage of peptide bonds involving tryptophan, especially at pH 4 to 5, probably due to spontaneous hydrolysis of the oxidole after cyclization to the iminolactone (Fig. 5.7). Oxidative cleavage of diiodotyrosyl-containing peptides has also been described. Modification of tryptophan residues during iodination at neutral or alkaline pH has been reported for lysozyme, casein, thyroglobulin, serum albumin, and gamma globulin. Tryptophan modifications on lysozyme are particularly apt to occur at positions 62 and 108, which are known to be exposed in the intact protein. Whether other amino acid residues are also oxidized is not presently known. α and β amino carboxylic acids have been shown to be oxidatively decarboxylated and deaminated by hypochlorite ions generated in the presence of chloramine T (Lambert and Jacquemin, 1973), but there is no evidence that this reaction occurs in intact proteins.

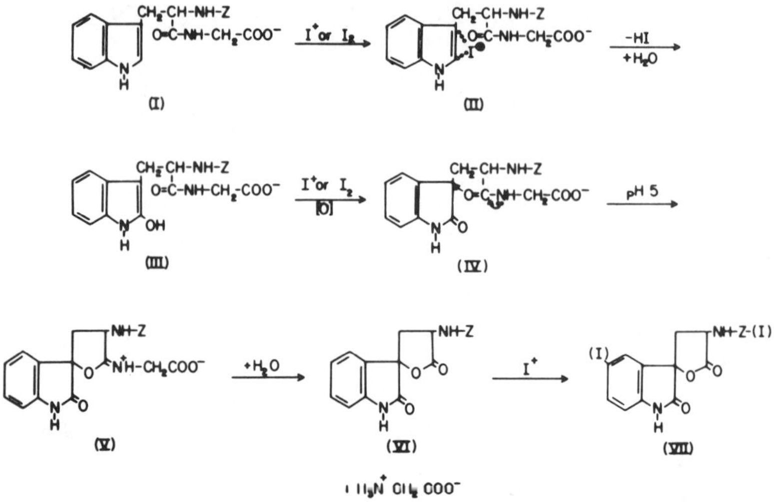

Fig. 5.7. Reaction mechanism for the oxidation and oxidative cleavage of a model tryptophane containing peptide during iodination. (Taken from N. M. Alexander. 1974. J. Biol. Chem. 249: 1946–1952.)

In addition to oxidative damage, the chemically reactive organic molecule chloramine T has the capacity of reacting directly with and substituting functional groups on proteins. This could well be a factor in the tendency of chloramine T-treated proteins to aggregate.

Fortunately, even with susceptible proteins, part of the available tyrosine groups are highly reactive, and levels of iodination consistent with the development of a practical radioimmunoassay can usually be obtained without undue oxidation or chloramine T substitution of the protein.

Denaturation. Denaturation during dilution, iodination, purification, and storage is a problem with some proteins. It can generally be predicted from the known behavior of the uniodinated protein in solution. If the stability of the protein is suspect, a blank iodination (without iodination reagents) can be used to detect damage of this kind. The maintenance of an appropriate ionic strength, divalent cation, or substrate concentration in the medium may help to prevent denaturation.

Impurities in the iodine. A practical and sometimes frustrating difficulty in iodination is a sporadic failure to obtain antigenically active or adequately iodinated products. Unsatisfactory preparations of iodinated antigen are obtained even by experienced investigators, utilizing iodination procedures that have been well standardized in their laboratories (Parker, 1972b). Most are probably due to undefined impurities in certain commercial lots of radioactive iodine. Products that have been observed in carrier-free preparations of ^{131} iodide, either before or after oxidation, include IO_3^-, IO_4^-, I^+, I_2, I_3, H_2O_2, IO_2^-, and free H and OH radicals (Cvoric, 1969). Unidentified radioiodine species are also present in some preparations. Problems in iodination are sporadically observed with both $^{125}I^-$ and $^{131}I^-$ regardless of the supplier and the extraction procedure used in preparing the radioiodine. Difficulties arise in all the commonly used iodination methods (Greenwood, 1971). Chloramine T oxidation is perhaps the most reliable of the various oxidation procedures, which helps explain its present popularity.

In addition to difficulties with fresh preparations of iodine, there may be problems with stored ^{125}I preparations that had been satisfactory for iodination purposes when first received. For this reason, many laboratories follow a procedure of never iodinating with iodine preparations that are more than 7 to 10 days old. Yet some preparations can be used successfully for much longer periods of time.

Decomposition during storage. Decomposition during storage of radiolabeled proteins is a serious problem with some proteins. Loss of antigenic reactivity with age is partly a reflection of radioactive decay with destruction of protein during emission of radioactivity. Dilution helps minimize the severity of the damage. As a rule, radioactive antigen preparations are diluted 10-to-100-fold in buffer containing an added protein (bovine serum albumin, egg albumin, gelatin, or diluted serum). Obviously the protein diluent must not cross-react immunologically with the antigen. The protein serves as a free-radical scavenger and may be helpful in other ways in avoiding damage during storage. Storage is usually in the frozen state, preferably at $-70°$. The work of Evans (1966) would suggest that there may be an additional advantage in storing preparations at liquid nitrogen temperature, since this appears to be useful with tritium-labeled compounds of high specific activity. It is common practice to freeze the diluted antigen in multiple, small airtight containers so that small volumes (0.2 to 0.3 ml) are thawed at a time and unused portions are not subjected to repeated freezing and thawing. The practical shelf life of the labeled antigen varies markedly with the protein, the extent to which it is labeled, and the sensitivity requirements of the assay. Often a stored preparation of antigen gives a less satisfactory assay from the point of view of assay sensitivity, variability, or susceptibility to nonspecific inhibition by tissue constituents. Alterations in radioactive antigen binding may be detected by a change in total marker binding or in the shape or sensitivity of the standard inhibition curve that is performed with each assay (Fig. 5.8). Flattening of the standard inhibition curve at low concentrations of unlabeled antigen is often the first alteration that is noticed. A fall in protein

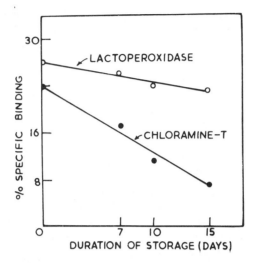

Fig. 5.8. Relative stability of iodinated FSH prepared by chemical and enzymatic methods. (Taken from N. R. Moudgal, and H. G. Madwha Raj. 1974. *In* B. M. Jaffe, and H. R. Behrman (Eds.). Methods of hormone radioimmunoassay. Academic Press, New York. pp. 57–85.)

immunoreactivity is frequently associated with protein denaturation and aggregation. As a rule, radioiodinated antigen preparations with suboptimal binding immediately after iodination show particularly rapid losses of binding, and it will eventually save time to reiodinate immediately. Sometimes a lot of radioiodinated antigen that is apparently comparable to earlier preparations will deteriorate rapidly during storage, for reasons that are not clear. Stored preparations with unfavorable binding curves can sometimes be used after further purification, shortly before use in the immunoassay (Fig. 5.9). For example, iodinated human-growth hormone retains high levels of immunoactivity for only a few days, but after repurification on a molecular sieve column, preparations that are several weeks old are suitable for immunoassay use.

Assessment of Iodination Damage

Some of the questions that may be considered in evaluating a radio-labeled antigen preparation are (a) the maximal percentage of antigen that is immunologically reactive (evaluated at high antibody concentrations), (b) the sensitivity and specificity of antigen binding under standard immunoassay conditions (at low antibody concentrations), and (c) the susceptibility of the iodinated antigen to changes in immunological reac-

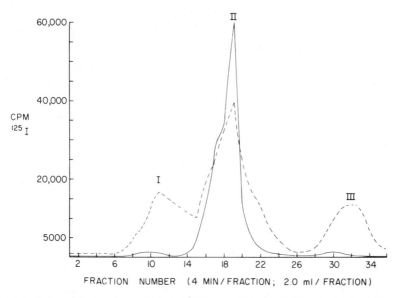

Fig. 5.9. Elution of fresh and stored labeled HGH from Sephadex G-100. On the day following iodination, nearly all the iodinated HGH was found in peak II, which is the most immunoreactive fraction (solid line). One month later there was a substantial increase in peaks I and III at the expense of peak II (dashed line). Peak I represents aggregated labeled growth hormone. Peak III is nonimmunoreactive. (Taken from G. T. Peake. 1974. In B. M. Jaffe, and H. R. Behrman (Eds.). Methods of hormone radioimmunoassay. Academic Press, New York. pp. 103–123.)

tivity during storage or incubation with tissue. If maximal antigen binding is all that is evaluated, relatively large amounts of antibody will be used, and subtle changes in antigen reactivity that might adversely affect assay sensitivity or specificity may remain undetected. Antigenic reactivity is therefore better assessed under operational immunoassay conditions, at limiting dilutions of antibody in the presence of graded amounts of un-labeled homologous, cross-reactive, and heterologous antigens, thus evaluating both for sensitivity and specificity of binding. The importance of subtle alterations in the antigen-binding curve will depend to a large extent on the sensitivity requirements of the assay. Although an undamaged tracer molecule is always desirable, the affinity of the labeled antigen need not be identical to that of the unlabeled antigen in order to have a workable assay. But if an extremely sensitive system is needed, seemingly minor alterations in antigen binding may result in an unsatisfactory assay. As discussed above, it may be helpful, in the initial evaluation of iodination damage, to use a lightly labeled antigen as a radioiodindicator molecule in order to evaluate damage in preparations of antigen exposed to graded amounts of duration reagents and ^{127}I. This step will distinguish reagent damage from damage associated with the physical introduction of iodine and will help identify an iodination condition that provides the best compromise between maximal specific activity and unacceptable antigenic damage. Another approach to detecting subtle changes in radiolabeled antigen binding is to see if the radioactive antigen and native (unexposed to iodination reagents) antigen have the same affinity for antibody. Various dilutions of antibody are incubated with radioactive antigen alone, at relatively high antigen concentrations, or with a mixture of radioactive and nonradioactive antigen at the same total antigen concentrations (e.g., 1.0 ng of ^{125}I antigen alone and 0.1 ng ^{125}I antigen mixed with 0.9 ng of unlabeled antigen; see Fig. 5.10 (Hunter, 1973). If the percentage of

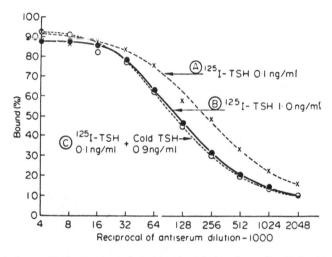

Fig. 5.10. Antiserum titration curves used to determine whether the marker binds with the same affinity to antibody as the unlabeled antigen. (Taken from W. M. Hunter. 1971. In K. E. Kirkham, and W. M. Hunter (Eds.). Radioimmunoassay methods. Churchill Livingstone, Edinburgh. pp. 3–23.)

bound radioactivity is the same with radiolabeled antigen alone as it is with the antigen mixture, we can assume that the labeled antigen has retained its affinity for antibody and that significant iodination damage has not occurred. When the label shows reduced binding affinity, there may be changes in some regions of the binding curve but not in others. Binding is more likely to be diminished at high ratios of total antigen to antibody, where competition between labeled and unlabeled antigen is maximized and species of antibody that are not of maximal affinity may be participating in binding. In this case, sensitivity may be improved by adjusting the antigen-antibody ratio.

Ways of Minimizing Iodination Damage or Effects of Iodination Damage in the Assay

USE OF DIFFERENT IODINATION REAGENTS

As noted, the use of lactoperoxidase or ICl has proved advantageous in proteins that are susceptible to chloramine T oxidation (see for example, Fig. 5.8). However, every one of the commonly used iodination procedures has drawbacks as well as advantages, and it is too much to expect that there would be a universal iodination procedure that gives superior results with every antigen. In the absence of detailed knowledge about antigen structure and reactivity, the problem can be approached empirically, beginning with chloramine T and lactoperoxidase and proceeding, if necessary, to other iodination methods or a systematic variation of the reaction conditions (see below). If satisfactory preparations are still not obtained, iodination of a carrier and secondary attachment to protein (see below) may be considered.

SYSTEMATIC MANIPULATION OF IODINATION CONDITIONS

Factors other than absolute tyrosine content exert a major influence on iodination. The susceptibility of individual protein tyrosyl groups to iodination varies with their microenvironment on the protein. Some tyroxyl groups are hydrogen bonded to nearby amino acids. Others are buried inside the protein, thus reducing their accessibility to the iodination reagents. The local environment may also influence the pK of the phenolic hydroxyl group of tyrosine. Not surprisingly, then, changes in the medium that affect protein conformation influence the iodination pattern obtained. Massaglia and his colleagues (1969) have studied the susceptibility of the four tyrosyl groups of insulin to iodination under a variety of experimental conditions. In aqueous solution from pH 1 to pH 9, iodination occurred primarily on tyrosyl groups of the A chain (presumably because of intramolecular hydrogen bonding in the B chain). Iodination in 8 M urea or in mixtures of water with organic solvents (ethylene glycol, propylene glycol, dioxane, ethanol, and methanol) resulted in a relative increase in uptake of iodine by B-chain tyrosyl groups. Observations with other proteins also indicate a hierarchy of reactivity with iodination of selected tyrosyls being favored, particularly under limiting iodination conditions (an unusually low iodination time or iodination reagent concentration). Thus, with some proteins at least, the iodination reactions can be manipulated so as to obtain substantial differences in the distribution of iodine.

The use of the lactoperoxidase or ICl methods may result in a different labeling pattern. Either approach may permit iodine groups to be directed away from areas that are critical for antigenic reactivity. However, selective iodination may not be possible with all proteins. The pattern of introduction of radioiodine into human-growth hormone differs markedly from that obtained with insulin (Hunter, 1967). Under standard iodination conditions radioiodine is introduced more or less evenly into the various tyrosyl residues on growth hormones, indicating that they are equally reactive. Whether there are other iodination conditions that would permit discriminatory tyrosyl labeling in this protein remains to be established.

IODINATION OF IMMUNOLOGICALLY COMPLEXED ANTIGEN
OR ANTIBODY

Another approach to obtaining partial selectivity of labeling is to iodinate in the presence of ligand. For example, an enzyme might be labeled in the presence of substrate in the hope that a configurational change associated with substrate binding would provide a more favorable distribution of iodine, thereby protecting its antigenic reactivity. This principle has been utilized in the iodination of antibodies. Antihapten antibodies frequently contain one or more tyrosyl groups in the combining sites, and in this case heavy iodination (usually more than five iodine atoms per molecule of protein) produces partial inactivation. When hapten is present, equally vigorous iodination results in considerably less inactivation, probably because tyrosyl residues in the combining region are less accessible to iodination reagents. Thus Koshland et al. (1962), working with rabbit antibenzenearsonate antibodies, found that the introduction of 3.6 atoms of iodine into the protein led to an 8% loss of total binding capacity, whereas 56 atoms of iodine led to an 88% loss of binding. However, when 53 atoms of iodine were introduced in the presence of hapten, the fall in binding was only 46%. Removal of the hapten and the introduction of only four more atoms of iodine (an increase from 53 to 57 atoms of iodine per molecule of protein) increased inactivation from 46 to 76%. Tyrosyl also appears to be present in the active site of anti-DNP antibodies. When anti-DNP antibodies were inactivated by iodination, peptide fractionation studies revealed that substitution of tyrosines in or near the combining site had occurred. Nonetheless, when anti-DNP or antibenzene-arsonate antibodies are *trace* labeled with iodine, binding activity is ordinarily well preserved even in the absence of hapten. Moreover, Johnson et al. (1966) studied a variety of antibodies and concluded that incorporation of less than two atoms of iodine resulted in no loss of activity. Thus unless unusually heavy iodination is required or the antibody is especially susceptible to inactivation, protection of the antibody-combining region is not necessary during iodination; it may even be undesirable, since removal of hapten after iodination may present difficulties.

Active-site protection may also be considered during iodination of antiprotein antibodies. Miles and Hales (1968) have advocated that anti-insulin antibody be iodinated while bound to insoluble insulin-cellulose in the expectation that a more reactive iodinated antibody would be obtained. However, they presented no direct evidence for protection; and it is important to emphasize that when other antiprotein antibodies have been *trace* labeled with iodine in the absence of antigen, satisfactory preparations have been obtained. By analogy with what has been observed with antihapten antibodies, protection of the combining site might be helpful for selected antibodies during heavy iodination. But heavy iodination may cause undesirable changes in the antibody molecule apart from binding-site inactivation per se and little would be gained.

It would also be possible to iodinate an antigen in the presence of insolubilized antibody and recover the antigen by a suitable dissociation procedure, which is the converse of the Miles and Hales procedure for obtaining radiolabeled antibody. Although this process might render antigenically reactive areas less accessible to iodination reagents, difficulties in eluting the antigen from the antibody and possible problems created by leakage of antibody from the absorbent would need to be considered. Certainly almost all proteins can be directly iodinated without resorting to a procedure of this kind. Nonetheless, the approach might prove to be useful for selected antigens and deserves systematic study.

ATTACHMENT OF IODINE TO PROTEIN THROUGH A CARRIER

The problem of iodination of antigenically important tyrosine residues can be avoided entirely by reacting the iodine with a suitable carrier first and then attaching the iodinated carrier to the protein. This method of iodination has the additional and potentially important advantage of avoiding the exposure of the protein to possible oxidation damage. The carrier can be a small molecular weight p-OH benzene derivative or a tyrosine-containing protein or polypeptide; 3-(p-hydroxylphenyl)-propionic acid-N-hydroxylsuccinimide (HPNS) has been used for this purpose (Bolton and Hunter, 1973; Hunter, 1974). HPNS has both a p-hydroxylphenyl group, making it easily iodinatable, and an active ester group, which gives it reactivity with nucleophilic amino acid residues on proteins. The HPNS is iodinated by the chloramine T procedure, extracted into benzene, and taken to dryness (Fig. 5.11). It is then reacted with the protein in aqueous solution at weakly alkaline pH. Peptide-bond formation takes place with protein amino groups, resulting in a stable attachment of radioactivity to the protein. Since the protein is not present during the iodination reaction, the method permits the iodination of proteins (or haptens) that are especially susceptible to damage during direct iodination. It can also be used

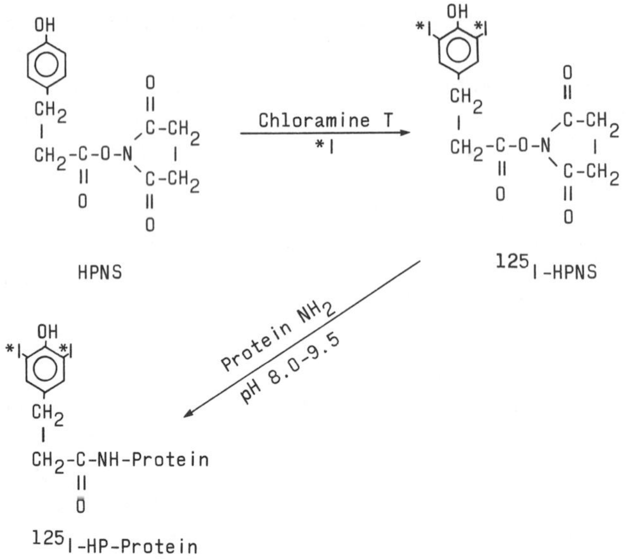

INDICATOR MOLECULES

Fig. 5.11. Steps in labeling a protein with iodinated hydroxyphenylpropionic acid N-hydroxy succinimide ester.

to iodinate proteins, polypeptides, or haptens that do not contain tyrosine but that do contain aliphatic amino groups, providing an alternative to introducing a phenolic group on the antigen prior to iodination. The use of HPNS avoids exposing the antigen to iodination reagents, but it does introduce a sizable organic molecule onto the protein with possible adverse effects on antigenic reactivity. The advantages and disadvantages of HPNS labeling will depend considerably on the protein. The use of HPNS has been reported to provide improved radioiodinated antigens in immunoassays for human-growth hormone and TSH (Hunter, 1974). However, these proteins were presumably selected because of their susceptibility to denaturation with conventional labeling procedures.

FRACTIONATION OF IODINATED ANTIGEN

Another approach to the problem of antigenic damage is to fractionate the iodinated antigen, the idea being to separate molecules of labeled protein that are immunologically inactive from those which retain their reactivity (Fig. 5.9). By choosing an appropriate chromatographic procedure, it may be possible to eliminate damaged protein at the same time that the unconjugated inorganic iodide is removed. For example, in preparing radiolabeled ACTH, it is desirable and convenient to remove degraded protein by chromatography on cellulose immediately after iodination. With small peptides, the charge differences between iodinated species are sufficient to separate monoiodinated from noniodinated or multi-iodinated peptides. This step may not be possible with sizable proteins because of the small contributions of iodotyrosine to overall protein charge (Landon et al., 1967). Another useful procedure is to absorb the radioiodinated antigen to insolubilized antibody and then elute with hapten or acid. Specific absorption, followed by elution, has been used with ^{125}I-labeled parathyroid hormone and angiotensin. It should, however, be noted that the presence of significant amounts of antigenically inactive protein, although always undesirable, does not necessarily cause major complications in the immunoassay, provided that the damaged protein does not bind nonspecifically.

Use of radioiodinated antibodies. For antigens that are unusually labile, it may be better to iodinate the antibody rather than the antigen, as discussed below.

Use of carefully chosen antisera. Freedlender and Cathou (1971) compared two anti-insulin antibodies, one of which reacted indistinguishably with insulin containing 0.5 to 2.7 iodine atoms/protein molecule, whereas the other bound progressively less insulin as the level of iodination was increased. The lack of parallelism between the two antisera could have been due to differences in specificity or affinity. The implications of this observation, in terms of how effects of iodination damage may be minimized in other systems, are obvious.

Radioiodinated Antibodies

So far it has been assumed that the antigen is radiolabeled rather than the antibody. Miles and Hales (1968) have pointed out possible advantages of using radioiodinated antibody as the marker. IgG, the predominant antibody in hyperimmune serum, contains numerous tyrosine residues and can be substituted with several iodine molecules without adverse effects on antibody activity. Iodination of antibody rather than antigen may be advantageous if the antigen is unusually susceptible to damage during iodination, storage, or incubation with tissue or if it lacks readily iodinatable residues. In the radioiodinated-antibody immunoassays, the antigen is attached to a solid-phase absorbant (Fig. 5.12). The antibody is radiolabeled with ^{125}I, usually after specific purification with antigen, to reduce or eliminate labeling of nonspecific gamma globulins. The method was applied initially to the immunoassay of bovine insulin (Miles and Hales, 1968).*

---

* Miles and Hales have applied the term *immunoradiometric* to this system. It is an unfortunate one, since, strictly speaking, all radioimmunoassays are immunoradiometric.

Diagram of the stages involved in the immunoradiometric assay

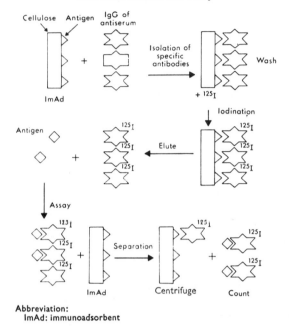

Abbreviation:
ImAd: immunoadsorbent

Fig. 5.12. Purification and iodination of antiinsulin antibodies on insulin-cellulose followed by elution and use of the iodinated antibodies in a quantitative sold-phase immunoassay for insulin. (Taken from J. S. Woodhead, G. M. Addison, and C. N. Hales. 1974. Brit. Med. Bull. 30:44–49.)

Guinea-pig anti-insulin antibody was specifically absorbed to an insulin-cellulose resin, radioiodinated in situ, and eluted with dilute acid. For the assay, purified ^{125}I-labeled antibody was reexposed to fresh insulin-cellulose in antigen excess in the presence and absence of free insulin. The radioactivity in the supernatant was shown to be a function of the concentration of soluble antigen. As little as 2 pg of insulin caused detectible inhibition of binding of the ^{125}I antibody to the resin.

The relative advantages and disadvantages of immunoassays that utilize radioiodinated antibodies are discussed in some detail in Chapter 6. Radioiodinated antibodies have been used in the measurement of insulin, parathormone, calcitonin, LH, FSH, growth hormone, angiotensin I, and ferritin, and apparently the procedure has general applicability. Useful applications outside the endocrine field have also been described. ^{125}I-anti-immunolobulin antibodies have been used to localize antigen binding to a specific immunoglobulin class. Excess insolubilized antigen is reacted sequentially with the unknown serum (containing an unspecified amount of first antibody) and with radiolabeled second antibody (specific for antigenic determinants on first antibody) (Wide et al., 1967). The first antibody binding is detected by an increase in radioactivity (second antibody) on the resin. This procedure has been used to determine antigen-binding activity in human IgE immunoglobulin (Fig. 5.13). Pollen antigens were

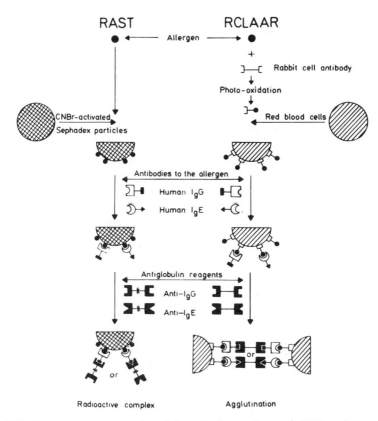

Fig. 5.13. Diagrammatic representation of the radioallergosorbent test (RAST) and the red-cell-linked antigen-antiglobulin reaction (RCLAAR). The RAST assay uses iodinated, antihuman IgE antibodies to detect IgE binding to antigen-containing particles. The RCLAAR assay uses agglutination as a measure of binding. (Taken from T. Berg, H. Bennich, and S. G. O. Johansson. 1971. Int. Arch. Allerg. 40:770–778.)

insolubilized on resin, exposed to sera from allergic and nonallergic individuals (in antigen excess), washed, and incubated with ^{125}I-labeled goat or rabbit anti-IgE antibodies. Human IgE antibodies specific for the resin-bound antigen were detected by an increase in ^{125}I radioactivity on the resin. The method can be used to determine small quantities of IgE antibodies in the presence of much larger quantities of IgM and IgG antibodies, although when the level of non-IgE antibodies is unusually high, antibody competition for antigenic determinants on the resin can occur. The specificity of the second antibody for immunoglobulin in question must, of course, be rigorously established or problems in interpretation could occur.

Proteins Labeled with Radioactive Markers Other than Iodine

Proteins and polypeptides have been labeled by acetylation with ^3H or ^{14}C acetic anhydride. Most of the reaction takes place with protein lysyl residues, although sulfhydryl, phenolic hydroxyl, and aliphatic hydroxyl groups can be substituted under appropriate conditions. The major drawback is that acetyl substitution on lysyl ϵ-ammonium groups causes a change in the charge properties of the protein with possible associated changes in antigenic reactivity, particularly at high levels of substitution (Fig. 5.14). And, unfortunately, a high substitution ratio may be needed to obtain a useful level of radioactivity, since the maximal specific activity of commercially available preparations of acetic anhydride is only 5 Ci/mmole (as compared with 2,500 Ci/mmole for commercially available ^{125}I). A better method for introducing ^3H involves

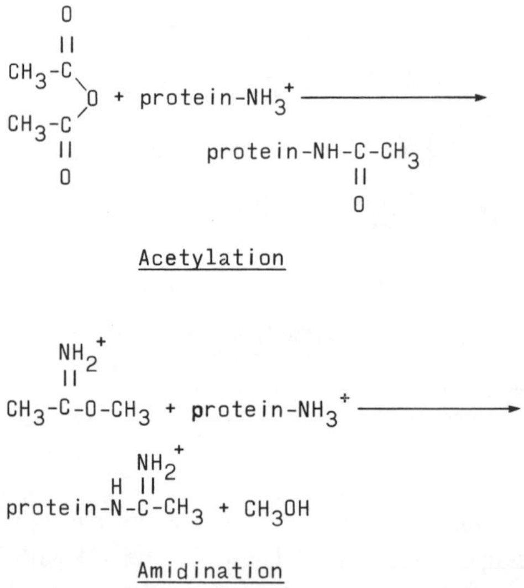

$$\begin{array}{c} O \\ \| \\ CH_3-C \\ \diagdown \\ \quad\quad O \;+\; \text{protein-NH}_3^+ \;\longrightarrow \\ \diagup \\ CH_3-C \\ \| \\ O \end{array} \quad\quad \text{protein-NH-C-CH}_3 \\ \quad\quad\quad\quad\quad\quad\quad\quad \| \\ \quad\quad\quad\quad\quad\quad\quad\quad O$$

Acetylation

$$\begin{array}{c} NH_2^+ \\ \| \\ CH_3-C-O-CH_3 \;+\; \text{protein-NH}_3^+ \;\longrightarrow \\ \\ \quad\quad\quad\quad NH_2^+ \\ \quad\quad H \; \| \\ \text{protein-N-C-CH}_3 \;+\; CH_3OH \end{array}$$

Amidination

Fig. 5.14. Comparative charge effects during acetylation and amidination of proteins. The reaction actually takes place with NH_2 groups on the protein, but NH_3^+ is shown to emphasize the fact that normally most of the amino groups are charged at neutral pH.

the use of labeled methyl acetimidate, which reacts specifically with lysyl and cysteinyl groups on proteins at pH 8.0 to 9.5, introducing an acetamidino group (Fig. 5.14). In contrast to acetic anhydride, when methyl acetimidate reacts with lysyl residues, it replaces the positive charge with another group of the same charge, and the isoelectric point of the protein is not altered. Indeed, more than 75% of the free amino groups of parathormone, insulin, or rabbit gamma globulin can be amidinated without demonstrable losses of hormonal or immunologic reactivity (Repke and Zull, 1972; Zull and Repke, 1972).

It seems probable that the introduction of ^{3}H or ^{14}C by amidination will be a useful adjunct to radioiodine labeling of antigens. The acetamidino group is less bulky than an iodotyrosine group, which could be an important advantage with some antigens. And since positively and negatively charged groups are likely to be located on the surfaces of proteins, whereas tyrosyl residues may be buried inside, destruction of protein conformation is perhaps less likely during amidination than during iodination (Repke and Zull, 1972). However, even by substituting all the free amino groups of insulin, the maximal specific activity obtained is only 36 Ci/mmole (9 Ci/mmole/free NH_2); and because of difficulties in preparing and storing maximally radioactive methyl acetimidate, the practical specific activity obtainable will probably be closer to 4 to 8 Ci/mmole protein (Repke and Zull, 1972). Thus, at best, the specific activities of amidinated proteins will be relatively low.

Labeling of protein can also be accomplished by an exchange with tritium gas by the Wilzbach procedure (Wilzbach, 1957), but the method may produce extensive denaturation and loss of antigenic reactivity, thereby requiring considerable repurification after labeling. Biosynthetically labeled proteins can be prepared, and, with efficient tissue culture systems and highly labeled amino acid precursors, relatively high specific activities can be obtained. Since intrinsically labeled proteins are not altered chemically, they have a theoretical advantage over radioiodinated proteins. However, only in rare cases would the improvement in antigenic reactivity warrant the increased preparative effort and probable reduction in specific activity. Moreover, if the protein is heavily labeled, deterioration during storage can be a serious problem, resulting in a shelf life that is little if any longer than that of an ^{125}I-labeled protein. Another way of labeling proteins involves an exchange reaction with tightly bound metals and enzymes. ^{63}Ni and ^{59}Fe have been used to label concanavalin A and iron-binding proteins, respectively, by this procedure. However, the label cannot be assumed to be completely stable, since there are heavy metals and enzymes in tissues that might displace or competitively bind the marker.

Various other radioactive molecules are also potentially usable as radioindicator molecules (e.g., ^{32}P or ^{35}S), but none has any special advantages over ^{125}I.

In summary, the advantages of using radioactive molecules other than radioiodine for labeling proteins and polypeptides are more imagined than real. In general, radioiodine can be introduced into antigen without major changes in immunologic reactivity or nonspecific binding, thus providing a convenient and sensitive radioindicator molecule. Even where initial iodination attempts give an unsatisfactory product, success may be achieved by altering the iodination conditions or prelabeling a carrier and attaching it to antigen. In unusual circumstances, the problems associated with iodination may be sufficiently vexing and the sensitivity requirements sufficiently low that the use of other radioactive markers may be desirable.

Radiolabeling of Macromolecules Other than Proteins

Nonprotein macromolecules like DNA or polysaccharides have been labeled biosynthetically, but this process is tedious (assuming that there is no commercial source) and the culture conditions required invariably place practical limitations on the specific activity that can be obtained. Terminal labeling is possible with ^{125}I, ^{3}H, or ^{14}C. Radioiodine has been introduced into polysaccharides by several methods. Ricketts (1966) labeled inulin and dextran by substituting an occasional allyl group into the molecule (by reaction with allyl bromide at alkaline pH with heating) and added radioiodine at the double bond. The radioiodine was introduced by converting it to free iodine in acid solution, but other iodination methods should be equally satisfactory. Although the resulting labeled alkyl iodide is an alkylating agent and can undoubtedly react with sulfhydryl and other groups on proteins, this type of label may be sufficiently stable for some immunoassay purposes. Siskind et al. (1967) prepared radioactively labeled pneumoccal polysaccharide S-III by alkylation of sugar OH groups with α-bromo-p-nitrotoluene, followed by reduction to p-OH-benzyl-S-III and introduction of ^{131}I by the chloramine T method. This procedure worked well with S-III polysaccharide, but the alkylation conditions were severe and may not be suitable for some polysaccharide antigens. Radioiodine can be incorporated into RNA and DNA at pH 5.0 in the presence of thallic trichloride (Scherberg and Refetoff, 1974). The reaction is largely specific for pyrimidine bases, although, under conditions of maximal labeling, limited substitution of adenine and guanosine is also obtained. A portion of the added iodine is spontaneously released, but if the iodinated nucleic acid is treated at alkaline pH for 20 minutes at 60°, the residual label is stable.

Double-stranded DNA has been labeled by complexing with radioactive actinomycin D, or by reaction with dimethyl sulfate, which is a methylating agent. Water-soluble carbodiimides can be labeled with tritium and used to form covalent bonds with purine and pyrimidine bases in DNA and RNA. Theoretically, a suitably substituted carbodiimide might be used to introduce a phenolic ring, which could then serve as a iodinatable residue in DNA and RNA.

Radioactive Haptens

Radioiodine has also been used as a marker in immunoassays involving haptenic determinants (Oliver et al., 1968; Parker, 1971). As a rule, this process involves the incorporation of a readily iodinatable group into the hapten. The hapten is first conjugated to tyrosine-containing protein or polyamino acid (or any derivative containing a p-hydroxyphenyl group). The use of imidazole groups as an iodinatable substituent may also be considered (Hunter, 1974). The development of a radioiodinated hapten for immunoassay purposes was first described for digitoxin (Oliver et al., 1966; Oliver et al., 1968; Parker, 1971). The aglycone of digitoxin was succinylated, coupled with tyrosine methyl ester, and iodinated. The marker could be used to measure serum levels of digitoxin, thus providing the first practical radioimmunoassay for a drug present at low concentrations in body fluids. Radioiodinated haptens have subsequently been used to measure cyclic AMP (Fig. 5.15), cyclic GMP, and testosterone. Because of the use of radioiodine in these markers, specific activities in excess of 150 Ci/mmole were readily obtained (Oliver et al., 1966; Steiner et al., 1969; Midgley et al., 1971). Although it might be assumed that the introduction of an iodinated benzene ring not represented on the immunogen would interfere with antibody binding, it has not been a problem, probably because the attachment to protein and to tyrosine was made at the same position on the hapten. Because of the hydrophobic properties of the aromatic ring carrying the iodine, the substitution may even aid in binding. Another strategy that might be followed is to attach the hapten to a tyrosine-containing protein or polypeptide carrier. This step permits the preparation of a radioiodinated, multivalent, hapten derivative (see Chapter 4 for a discussion of possible effects on sensitivity). If the haptenic portion of the hapten-protein conjugate is stable, the coupling and iodination conditions can be relatively severe, since there is no need to preserve the antigenic reactivity of the protein itself

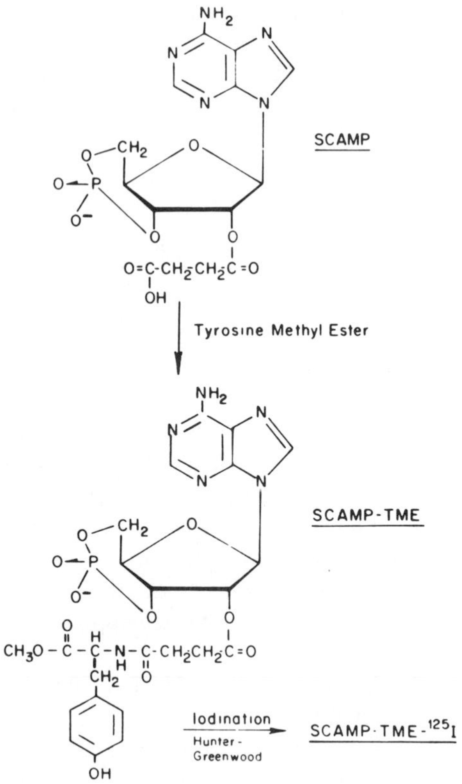

Fig. 5.15. Synthesis and iodination of a tyrosine derivative of cAMP (SCAMP-TME) for use as a radioindicator molecule in the cAMP immunoassay. The coupling agent is N,N'-dicyclohexylcarbodiimide (DCC). (Taken from A. L. Steiner, C. W. Parker, and D. M. Kipnis. 1970. *In* P. Greengard and E. Costa (Eds.). Advances in biochemical psychopharmacology. Vol. 3. Raven Press, New York. pp. 89–111.)

and a protein can be chosen that will give a limited degree of nonspecific binding. If hapten-protein conjugates are used for iodination, it is important to observe the precaution of choosing another protein and coupling agent than the ones used in preparing the immunizing antigen. Otherwise antibodies to the protein or coupling agent could cause problems in interpretation in the immunoassay (Goodfriend et al., 1964; Halloran and Parker, 1966). Polypeptides in which no tyrosine is present can also be conjugated to proteins and polyaminoacids that contain tyrosyl groups in order to obtain an antigen that can be iodinated. Iodinated derivatives of bradykinin (Goodfriend and Ball, 1969) and gastrin tetrapeptide (Newton et al., 1970) have been obtained in this way, thereby avoiding the laborious process of totally synthesizing polypeptide analogs in which an antigenically, noncritical amino acid residue is replaced by tyrosine. Another procedure that can be used with polypeptides is to attach a single p-hydroxyphenyl group to the N-terminal or C-terminal end of the molecule; Goodfriend and Ball (1969) reacted the o-nitrophenyl ester of desaminotyrosine with the α-amino group of bradykinin and obtained a bradykinin derivative that could be easily iodinated.

Problems arise in developing a radioiodine marker for a haptenic system when the hapten is altered chemically during iodination. For example, morphine and its congeners are highly susceptible to oxidation, and up to the present time ^{14}C and ^{3}H markers have been used even though the synthesis of a tyrosine derivative of morphine does not present serious difficulties. Oxidation is also a problem in preparing radioiodinated prostaglandin markers, although there is evidence that, in polyaminoacids containing both prostaglandin and tyrosine, useful amounts of radioactivity can be incorporated without an overriding loss of immunoreactivity (Levine and Van Vunakis, 1970). Therefore before attempting to synthesize a tyrosyl that contains hapten, it is important to consider the question of hapten susceptibility to oxidation. This factor can often be predicted from the known chemical properties of the hapten or may be assessed directly by exposing the unmodified hapten to [127]I and various iodination reagents and evaluating for changes in chromatographic or immunologic activity (changes in immunologic reactivity are detected by a diminution in its ability to inhibit the reaction between antibody and ^{3}H-or ^{14}C-labeled hapten). Difficulties due to direct damage to the hapten in iodinating mixtures can be circumvented by iodinating a phenolic hydroxyl-containing compound first and then coupling it to the hapten. A suitable molecule, 3-(p-hydroxyphenyl) propionic acid-N-hydroxysuccinimide ester (Bolton and Hunter, 1973), is discussed in the section on protein labeling. The major disadvantages of this procedure are the increased number of manipulations required and the possible practical limitations that may exist on the specific activity of the final product. Whenever possible, direct iodination is preferable. Under ordinary circumstances radioiodinated haptens are greatly preferred over ^{3}H-or ^{14}C-labeled haptens in routine immunoassays. By using iodinated haptens, the expense and time involved in preparing samples for liquid scintillation counting, as well as the longer counting times needed to obtain comparable levels of sensitivity, can be avoided. When dealing with structurally complex haptens having numerous potential sites for the introduction of ^{3}H or ^{14}C, the difference in specific activity is less marked than it is with haptens of molecular weight less than 300. Moreover, the bulk, hydrophobicity, and negative charge of the iodophenol moiety may result in increased nonspecific binding to glassware or other components of the incubation mixture. In this event, a time-consuming extraction procedure may be required if a ^{125}I marker is used, and a ^{3}H or ^{14}C marker may actually be preferable. The likelihood that an iodinated marker will exhibit high nonspecfic binding is increased if the unsubstituted hapten itself is subject to nonspecfic binding. However, if ^{3}H-and ^{14}C-labeled haptens of high specific activity are used, careful attention is needed in regard to the stability of the marker during storage.

Procedures for separating hapten-iodotyrosine conjugates from free ^{125}I differ from the ones used in purifying iodinated proteins because of the smaller molecular weight of the hapten, which may preclude separation on Sephadex G-25. Thin-layer chromatography or gel filtration of Sephadex G-10 or Biogel P-2 can be used instead. Radioiodinated haptens may adhere to Sephadex G-10, and the elution pattern cannot always be predicted on the basis of molecular size alone (Steiner et al., 1969).

Nonradioactive Indicator Molecules

Enzyme Immunoassays

It is possible to carry out competitive binding assays by using non-radioactive markers. One approach is to conjugate an antibody or antigen to an enzyme and measure binding by following changes in enzymatic activity—in effect, using catalytic activity in place of radioactivity. A stable enzyme, easily attached to antigen or antibody, with a high turnover number is required. The enzyme should not be unduly subject to interference in the presence of tissue, serum, or extracts, and a convenient, rapid, and sensitive means of measuring substrate hydrolysis should be available. Success has been attained in the measurement of polypeptide hormones and estrogens with antigens conjugated to alkaline phosphatase or horseradish peroxidase, utilizing a chromogeneic or fluorogenic substrate (Van Weemen and Schuurs, 1972). The experience is already extensive enough to indicate that enzyme assays will be applicable to almost any antigen-antibody system.

A particularly interesting enzyme immunoassay involves an ability of antihapten antibodies to change the activity of hapten-substituted enzymes. In previous studies with antienzyme antibodies, enzyme activity could be enhanced or inhibited, presumably because of a favorable or unfavorable change in the conformation of the enzyme catalytic site in the presence of antibody. Rubenstein et al. (1972) extended this principle to hapten-substituted enzymes (Fig. 5.16). They found that when purified chicken lysozyme was substituted with morphine and anti-morphine antibody was added, the enzyme was inactivated. Free hapten was able to prevent the inactivation at sufficiently low concentrations to

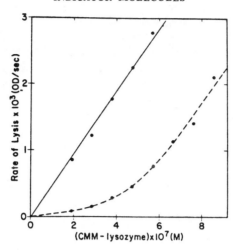

Fig. 5.16. Rate of lysis of *M. luteus* by carboxymethyl morphine-substituted lysozyme in the presence – – – – and absence ———— of antimorphine γ-globulin (4.2 x 10^{-7} M binding sites). (Taken from K. E. Rubenstein, R. S. Schneider, and E. F. Ullman. 1972. Biochem. Biophys. Res. Commun. 47:846–851.)

provide a practical immunoassay. Using lysozome as the indicator enzyme, the alteration in enzyme activity can be monitored by following changes in the turbidity of the solution through an insoluble substrate. The assay should be applicable to virtually any hapten, although a careful choice of conjugation conditions may be needed to ensure that the enzyme is not irreversibly inactivated by the hapten-substitution reaction per se. As in the fluorescence polarization and electron spin resonance procedures (see below), there is the advantage that separation of bound from free hapten is not necessary in determining binding. This fact simplifies the assay to the point that it can be used for rapid screening in the absence of elaborate equipment (see discussion below under fluorescence polarization).

Conventional enzyme immunoassays, as presently applied, have not had any important advantage over radioimmunoassays in terms of sensitivity and specificity. Indeed, in the haptenated lysozyme immunoassay, sensitivity is five- or tenfold less than that of a conventional radioimmunoassay using ^{14}C- or ^{3}H-dihydromorphine as a marker. Of course, if the elegant enzyme-recycling techniques of Lowry (Lowry and Passonneau, 1972) are used, the sensitivity of the enzyme measurement could be extended to the point that the only limitation on immunoassay sensitivity would be antibody affinity. But the number of manipulations and possible sources of error would also be increased. One area where enzyme immunoassays might be of particular value would be in the development of immunoassay kits for emergency medical diagnosis (e.g., in the use of immunoassays for bacterial antigen detection, as is desirable in the diagnosis of acute meninigitis). Since sensitive fluorometric instruments are relatively inexpensive, it would be financially feasible to equip even small laboratories for fluorometric enzyme immunoassays.

Fluorescence Polarization

Fluorescence polarization measurements can also be used to follow antigen reactions. If an antigen of reasonably low molecular weight (less than 40,000) is conjugated with fluorescein or some other suitable fluorescent molecule and reacted with antibody, a change in fluorescence polarization will be observed (Parker, 1973). The binding of a small protein molecule to antibody decreases its rate of movement in solution, thus increasing the polarization of fluorescence (Fig. 5.17). The method

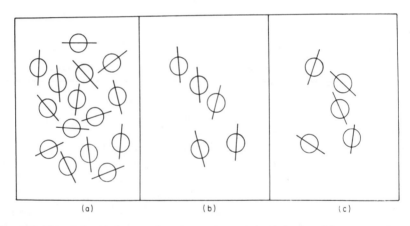

(a)   (b)   (c)

Fig. 5.17. The relationship between Brownian motion and depolarization of fluorescence. Protein molecules in solution are represented by ϕ. As shown in (a) they are randomly oriented. Excitation by polarized light preferentially excites molecules lying parallel to one another (b). By the time fluorescence is emitted (c), excited molecules have become partially but not completely disoriented, and the fluorescence is partially polarized. If the fluorescence of free hapten is measured (not shown), movement is so rapid that there is no polarization. However, if the hapten is bound to protein, partial polarization is seen, just as it is with the protein itself. (Taken from G. Weber. 1953. Advances Protein Chem., 8:415–459.)

is applicable to proteins and polypeptides, the magnitude of the change in polarization increasing as the size of the fluorescent molecule is decreased. The change in polarization develops over a period of 5 to 10 minutes, reflecting the time required to approach maximal binding.

Haptens attached to fluorescein groups may also be used, provided that the linkage between the two molecules does not permit too much free rotation. In some systems the sensitivity of the method approaches that of a radioimmunoassay. The most important theoretical advantage of the system is that bound and free antigen can be measured together, thereby eliminating the need for a separation procedure. One drawback is the possibility of nonspecific interactions between the fluorescent marker and serum or tissue proteins complicating the interpretation of the binding. Moreover, protein fluorescence or light scattering (in turbid samples) may increase fluorescence blanks to the point that the theoretical sensitivity of the method is not realized. Neither limitation is insurmountable. Although it seems doubtful that polarization measurements will supercede radioimmunoassays to any major extent, useful applications can be anticipated. In particular, the possibility of making rapid measurements of antigen binding without separating bound and free antigen by using easily portable fluorometric equipment would suggest that the method would be of value for rapid screening under field conditions (see enzyme section immunoassay).

Electron Spin Resonance

Another interesting approach to the immunoassay of small molecular weight haptens is the use of electron spin resonance (ESR). In this technique the hapten is attached to a stable, organic, free radical, usually a nitroxide. Nitroxides have a characteristic sharp-banded electron spin resonance spectrum during electronic perturbation in aqueous solution. When the haptenic group interacts specifically with antibody, the nitroxide radical is largely immobilized and a broadened ESR pattern is obtained. The change in the ESR signal can be used to quantitate the antibody-hapten reaction, and, as in other immunoassay procedures, unlabeled hapten inhibits the change. Initially ESR was used to study model antibody-hapten interactions using antibodies specific for the DNP group (Stryer and Griffith, 1965; Hsia and Piette, 1969). Subsequently, ESR has been applied to the detection of morphine in serum by Leute et al. (1972; Leute, 1973) using antibodies to 3-carboxymethyl-morphine and a carboxymethyl-morphine nitroxide derivative (Fig. 5.18). The beauty of the method lies in its simplicity and rapidity. If the hapten and spin-labeled hapten do not interact nonspecifically with serum proteins, the assay can be applied directly to serum as an essentially instantaneous method of measuring binding. Unfortunately, with present instrumentation, the sensitivity of the method is at several orders of magnitude below

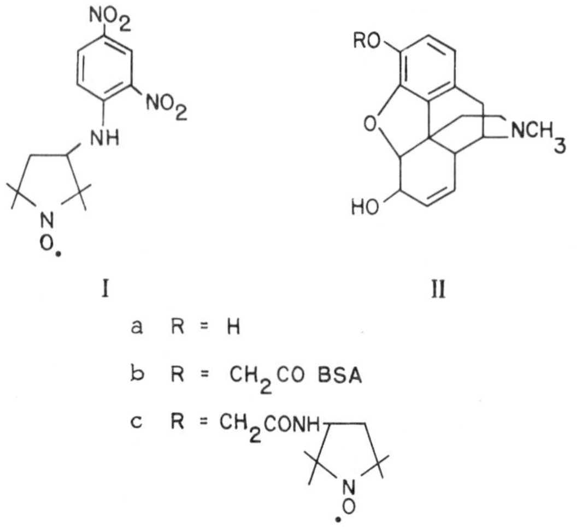

I   II

    a   R = H

    b   R = CH₂CO BSA

    c   R = CH₂CONH

Fig. 5.18. Electron spin resonance markers on DNP (I) and morphine (IIc). Morphine itself is IIa, and the immunogen for preparing the antimorphine antibody is IIb. (Taken from R. K. Leute, E. F. Ullman, A. Goldstein; and L. A. Herzenberg. 1972. Nature New Biol. 236:93–94.)

that of conventional radioimmunoassays. And the nature of the change in the ESR signal during binding is such that precise quantitation of bound and free marker is difficult. Moreover, careful temperature control is needed to avoid misinterpretation caused by temperature effects on the ESR signal (Copeland, 1973). If the sensitivity and precision can be improved, the method will probably come into widespread clinical use in rapid screening for drugs that circulate in the blood at concentrations in the intermediate concentration range.

Other Methods

A variety of other methods can be applied to the measurement of antigen, including phage neutralization, hemagglutination (Fig. 5.13) or neutralization of the biologic activity of the antigen. Phage-neutralization immunoassays are based on the ability of specific antibody to react a hapten- or protein-substituted phage and interfere with its ability to replicate in tissue culture. Because a single molecule of antibody is theoretically capable of neutralizing an entire particle of phage, the method is very sensitive (to 10^{-5} to 10^{-6} μg of antigen). Unfortunately, it is much too cumbersome for routine use. Hemagglutination inhibition is useful as a rapid and sensitive screening procedure for an antigen but is less quantitative and reproducible than other methods.

Summary

1. Almost all immunoassays utilize an easily measured indicator molecule, attached either to the antigen or the antibody, as a means of following the antigen-antibody reaction. Ordinarily the antigen rather than the antibody is labeled.

2. Useful indicator systems include radioactivity, enzymatic activity, fluorescence, and electron spin resonance.

3. As a rule, radioactive indicator molecules are used, and of these ^{125}I has been the most satisfactory.

4. Radioiodine is readily introduced into tyrosine-containing proteins by chemical (chloramine T or iodine monochloride) or enzymatic (lactoperoxidase) oxidation. Under appropriate conditions iodine can also be introduced onto histidyl or cysteinyl residues.

5. The optimal iodination procedure must be determined empirically for each antigen, attempting to find the maximal level of label that can be incorporated without reducing immunologic reactivity or otherwise significantly altering the physicochemical properties of the molecule adversely. In general, the optimal level of labeling is about one iodine atom/ molecule of protein. Attempts to increase the level of iodination further, while theoretically desirable from the point of permitting shorter counting times or small incubation volumes, normally do not yield major increases in sensitivity because antibody affinity and experimental variability become limiting. Even when a satisfactory iodination procedure has been evolved, each new labeled antigen preparation must be screened carefully, both initially and after storage, for damage that would adversely affect assay sensitivity, specificity, reproducibility, or usability in tissue extracts.

6. Although the basis for iodination damage to antigenic reactivity is incompletely understood, aggregation, oxidation, alterations in overall charge, and substitution of iodine onto critical amino acid residues in antigenically important areas all appear to be involved.

7. If iodination damage to the antigen turns out to be a major problem, possible approaches include (a) use of a different iodination method (enzymatic iodination has been shown to be preferable to chemical iodination for a number of highly sensitive proteins); (b) a systematic manipulation of iodination conditions; (c) iodination of antigen-antibody complexes rather than free antigen; (d) introduction of iodine via a carrier so that the protein is never directly exposed to the iodination reagents; (e) removal of damaged iodinated antigen fractions by selective absorption or chromatography; (f) introduction of the radiolabel onto the antibody rather than the antigen; and (g) careful selection of antisera that have minimal susceptibility to iodination damage of the antigen.

8. Iodinated, specifically purified antibodies can be used in conjunction with insolubilized, unlabeled antigens for immunoassay measurements. This method has certain theoretical advantages, particularly if the antigen is easily damaged by iodination but has not been rigorously compared, in terms of sensitivity and reproducibility, with labeled antigen methods. Using a radiolabeled second antibody and unlabeled first antibody, the method can be used to determine the quantity of first antibody belonging to a specific immunoglobulin class.

9. Proteins can be labeled with radioactive markers other than iodine. The use of ^{3}H methyl or ethyl acetimidate may be considered if iodination damage is a problem and high specific activity is not needed.

10. Although nucleic acids, polysaccharides, and lipids can be labeled biosynthetically, methods for introducing extrinsic labels after biosynthesis are now being developed. As radiolabeled preparations of higher specific activity become available, more sensitive procedures for measuring these substances will almost certainly evolve.

11. Haptens are usually labeled either with ^{125}I or with ^{3}H. With small haptens, the use of ^{125}I has major advantages because of the large potential gain in specific activity. The advantage is less marked with large, structurally complex haptens because higher levels of ^{3}H specific activity (on a molar basis) are achievable. As a rule, radioiodine is introduced onto the hapten through a p-hydroxyphenyl group. The p-hydroxyphenyl group is attached covalently to the hapten and iodinated by using a conventional protein-iodination reagent.

12. Particle aggregation (agglutination or flocculation), fluorescent, enzymatic, and electron spin resonance immunoassays can also be used. Many of them eliminate the need to separate free and bound antigen and thereby lend themselves to rapid screening. However, depending on the method, they may suffer from lack of sensitivity, precision, or reproducibility. Enzymatic methods for measuring the labeled antigen could, theoretically, be made a great deal more sensitive (by use of enzyme recycling techniques), but doing so would not necessarily increase assay sensitivity or precision to any major extent, since antibody affinity and experimental errors inherent in establishing the competitive binding reaction and separating free and bound antigen would then become limiting.

Chapter 6

The Immunoassay. Thermodynamic and Kinetic Considerations

ANTIBODY AFFINITY AND AVIDITY

Antibody-Hapten Interactions

As noted earlier, antibody affinity can vary over a broad range, resulting in marked variations in assay sensitivity. The importance of antibody affinity in hapten binding can be illustrated by a simple calculation. In the law of mass action

$$(1) \qquad K_a = \frac{(Ab \cdot H)}{(Ab)(H)}$$

Under conditions in which 50% of the total hapten is antibody bound, $Ab \cdot H = H$, and the equation reduces to

$$(2) \qquad K_a = \frac{1}{(Ab)}$$

In other words, the concentration of free antibody that must be maintained in order to bind 50% of the hapten is inversely proportional to K_a. In a competitive radioimmunoassay, it is not always necessary to achieve 50% binding of marker (although this amount is often what is used), but binding cannot be much less than 25% or the level of bound radioactivity will be too small. As an initial approximation, then, the K_a of the antibody determines the maximal dilution of antiserum that can be used to obtain adequate binding of marker. And if a high concentration of antibody is needed, the ability of small quantities of unlabeled hapten to compete with marker for antibody is decreased, thereby lowering the sensitivity of the assay. Thus if the association constant of the antibody is 1×10^6 liters/mole, the concentration of antibody required to obtain 50% antigen binding will be about 1×10^{-6} M (approximately 80 μg antibody protein/ml),

111

and the sensitivity of the assay will be in the high nanomole to low micio-mole range. But if the K_a is above 1×10^8 liters/mole, the sensitivity of the assay can extend into the picomole range. As noted, experimentally, K_a's ranging between 5×10^4 and 1×10^{11} liters/mole^{-1} have been reported. The highest K_a values for haptens have been obtained with bulky, hydrophobic molecules (such as digitoxin, digoxin, dansyl, and DNP) or molecules with multiple charged groups in addition to large hydrophobic regions (dichlorofluorescein). For most antihapten antibodies, average association constants are in the range of 10^5 to 10^7 liters/mole^{-1}, which may or may not be adequate for immunoassay purposes, depending on the sensitivity and on whether a subpopulation of higher-affinity antibodies is also present. As suggested in an earlier section, some haptens probably lack the structural complexity and molecular bonding properties required to produce high-affinity antibodies.

Antibody-Protein Interactions

Affinity also has an important influence on antigen-antibody reactions involving proteins and antiprotein antibodies, although the mathematical treatment is more complicated because of the multivalence and structural complexity of the antigen. Unless the antigen or antibody is univalent, lattice formation occurs, thus making it impossible to obtain a true affinity value for the interaction of antibody with individual antigenic determinants. What is being measured is the overall avidity of a mixture of different antibodies for the protein as a whole, which, under equilibrium conditions, may be as much a product of secondary aggregation as it is of primary binding. Protein-antiprotein interactions may also result in precipitation and associated changes in free energy as protein molecules are transferred from solution into a solid phase, thus further complicating the analysis (Karush, 1962).

Although the available data are less extensive for protein than for haptenic determinants, it is clear that the stability of the association between antibodies and multivalent protein antigens varies over a broad range, just as it does with antibodies and haptens. Using fluorescence polarization measurements, Dandliker and de Saussure (1970) obtained average association K_{avid} (avidity)* constants of 2×10^8 liters/mole^{-1}

---

* The term *avidity* will be applied to the overall stability of complexes formed between multivalent antigens and multivalent antibody molecules, the word *affinity* being restricted to interactions between monovalent ligands and single antibody-combining sites (Eisen, 1966).

for rabbit antiovalbumin and rabbit antibovine serum albumin. By radio-immunoassay, avidity constants in the range of 10^{12} to 10^{13} liters/mole^{-1} have been calculated for antibodies to several peptide hormones (insulin, ACTH, and gastrin; Yalow and Berson, 1971). These extremely high values help explain why low picogram quantities of protein can sometimes be detected by radioimmunoassay.

The Role of Antigen Valence in Stabilization of Immune Complexes

MONOGAMOUS BIVALENT BINDING

The high-avidity values in selected antibody peptide, or antibody-protein interactions reflect, at least in part, the ability of sizable peptides and proteins to interact with multiple antibody molecules simultaneously. The role of antigen valence in stabilizing antigen-antibody complexes is well illustrated in a study by Hornick and Karush (1969) with DNP-substituted bacteriophage. The bacteriophage was reacted with DNP-sulfonate, which substitutes lysyl residues on the phage with DNP. Under equilibruim conditions the hapten-substituted phage was inactivated by anti-DNP antibody (obtained by immunization with DNP-bovine gamma globulin) with an inactivation constant (K_I) of 3.5×10^{11} mole^{-1}. On the basis of the kinetics of inactivation, it was concluded that inactivation could be achieved by the binding of one antibody molecule at a single critical site on the phage, which means that the inactivation constant should be a good approximation of the K_a. By equilibrium dialysis, the same antibody was found to have a K_a for ϵ-DNP-lysine of only 6×10^6 liter/mole^{-1}, more than four orders of magnitude below its K_I for the DNP-substituted phage. The most probable cause of the energetic advantage in the reaction of antibodies with phage is the multivalence of the phage. This feature permits a single antibody molecule to attach to two haptenic groups on the same phage particle (monogamous bivalent binding), thereby stabilizing the interaction and increasing the effective affinity. An analogous cooperative binding effect in which a single molecule of antibody is bound at two sites on a protein is theoretically possible in antibody interactions with soluble proteins containing paired or multiple antigenic determinants. This type of binding may also occur with polysaccharides, polyamino acids, or nucleic acids, where the same antigenic determinant is repeated many times on the same molecule of polymer. Since the relationship between the two combining sites on a single molecule of IgG antibody is largely fixed, the ability of the antibody to react bivalently with a single molecule of polymer is importantly influenced by the fine structure and flexibility of the polymer. Two of the most critical factors are the frequency and spacing of the determinant.

MULTAGAMOUS BIVALENT BINDING

Another form of stabilization is obtained when antibodies form multiple bridges between antigen molecules (multagamous bivalent binding). The extent of bridging will depend on the number and distribution of immunologically reactive areas on the antigen, its overall size and charge, and the affinity and fine specificity of the antibody. If the antigen is a sizable protein, there is no reason why four or five antibody molecules of different specificities could not be attached to the same antigen molecule, thus stabilizing the complex.

ATTEMPTS TO MAXIMIZE ANTIGEN VALENCE
IN PROTEIN-ANTIPROTEIN INTERACTIONS

In general, we might expect that, as valence of antigen is increased, binding and cross linking of antigen molecules by antibody would also increase, thereby augmenting the sensitivity of the system. Therefore one of the goals of immunization may be to produce an antiserum that recognizes as many independent domains on the antigen as possible. Metzger (1967) has pointed out that because the antibody response to a protein is normally heterogeneous, the number of different antibody specificities that are obtained in a single antiserum is increased, which amplifies the effective valence of the antigen. Since antigen valence is affected by the mode of immunization and the time at which sera are harvested, part of what is accomplished by hyperimmunization with proteins, polypeptides, or structurally complex haptens may be to maximize the diversity of antibody specificities present in the serum. As noted, species differences also influence the number of determinants recognized on the antigen. In obtaining antibodies to protein or polypeptide hormones, the more foreign the protein is, the greater the likelihood that it will differ from the host protein at multiple sites and produce antisera that see the antigen as being multivalent. If maximization of antigen valence is indeed advantageous for increasing sensitivity, we might expect that, in selected immunoassay systems involving complex antigens, properly chosen mixtures of antisera obtained from the same or different animal species would give more sensitive immunoassays than sera from individual animals. As far as we know, this question has not been systematically studied. It is possible that attempts to utilize as many antigenic specificities as possible by the use of pooled antisera would result in competition of antibodies for overlapping areas of the protein or an unacceptable level of immunologic cross-reactivity.

THE USE OF MULTIVALENT HAPTEN MARKERS

Because of the operational increase in affinity when antibodies interact with multivalent antigens, the question arises as to whether hapten immunoassay sensitivity would be improved by using a multivalent radioindicator molecule. Normally this process would be accomplished by substituting the hapten more or less randomly on a multifunctional protein or polypeptide. Indeed, if desired, hapten molecules might be spaced on a carefully selected carrier so as to favor a bivalent attachment of antibody to adjacent hapten groups on the same molecule of carrier. It might also be possible to polymerize the antibody, increasing its valence while attempting to avoid major changes in nonspecific binding. Radioindicator molecules in which multiple haptenic groups are attached to an iodinated carrier have been used in immunoassays for penicilloyl antibodies (Thiel et al., 1964) and prostaglandin, morphine, and gastrin tetrapeptide antigens (Newton et al., 1970; Levine et al., 1971; Van Vunakis et al., 1972), but no convincing evidence has been presented that assay sensitivity is substantially improved. The major difficulty is that as the stability of the antibody-multivalent ^{125}I antigen complex is increased, molecules of unknown univalent hapten become less capable of competing with the marker. Thus either an increase or a decrease in assay sensitivity is theoretically possible as the valence of the antigen is increased. Levine et al. (1971) reported that the sensitivity of immunoassay measurements for monovalent prostaglandins was no better using an ^{125}I-labeled, multivalent, prostaglandin polyamino acid conjugate marker than a univalent ^{3}H prostaglandin marker. Our own unpublished studies in the same system indicated that the univalent ^{3}H prostaglandin marker was actually preferable, in terms of both assay sensitivity and specificity * (Jaffe and Parker, unpublished observations). With selected haptens, the diminution in competitive effectiveness might theoretically be circumvented by polymerizing or otherwise altering the unknown hapten in situ. In at least one haptenic system it has been possible to alter the unknown hapten in tissue extracts chemically, thereby increasing its structural similarity to the haptenic group on the immunogen. Thus in radioimmunoassay measurements for cyclic AMP, assay sensitivity can be increased up to a hundredfold by quantitatively converting cAMP in the unknown sample to 2'O-succinyl-cyclic AMP by reaction with excess succinic anhydride in weakly alkaline aqueous solution (Cailla et al., 1973) (Fig. 6.1). Succinyl cAMP is better able to compete in the cAMP radioimmunoassay than unaltered cAMP

---

* Oxidation of the cyclopentane ring on a portion of the conjugated prostaglandin residues is theoretically possible during iodination and could have influenced the binding results above.

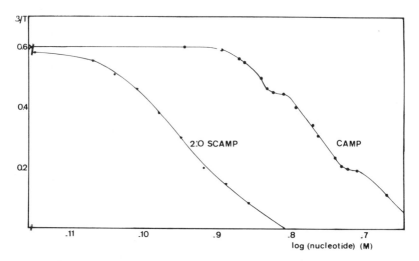

Fig. 6.1. Displacement of iodinated succinyl cAMP tyrosine methyl ester marker (^{125}I-SCAMP-TME, see legends to Figs. 1.1 and 5.15) from antibody by 2'0-succinyl cAMP and cAMP. The data are plotted as the ratio [bound [125]ISCAMPTME]/[bound + free [125]ISCAMPTME] (ordinate) versus log [nucleotide]. (Taken from H. L. Cailla, M. S. Racine-Weisbuch, and M. A. Delaage. 1973. Anal. Biochem. 56:394-407.)

because both the immunogen (a 2'O-succinyl-cyclic AMP-protein con-jugate) and the marker (a 2'O-succinyl-tyrosine-methyl ester derivative of cyclic AMP that has been iodinated) contain the succinyl group, and succinyl cyclic AMP is therefore the homologous hapten (see Fig. 2.7). The major drawback to chemical alterations of the unknown hapten is the increase in the number of manipulations, which increases the time re-quired to process samples and quite possibly decreases the reproductibility of the assay. Another way to minimize the diminution in competitive effectiveness when a univalent hapten competes with a multivalent marker is to utilize a nonequilibrium assay (see below). The antibody is pre-incubated with hapten in the tissue sample and then allowed to react with the multivalent marker for a limited period of time. The usefulness of this approach is determined by the ability of the unknown hapten to remain associated with antibody over the time period required to achieve an efficient, high-affinity association of the marker with the antibody (see below).

Unequal Competition of Unlabeled Antigen and
Antigen Marker for Antibody

From the preceding discussion it is apparent that any increase in the operational avidity of the antibody-marker interaction is of little or no value if the inhibitory potency of the unknown hapten in the system is correspondingly decreased. The relative inhibitory capacity of the unlabeled hapten is just as important with univalent as with multivalent markers. In the cAMP immunoassay example given, succinylation of cAMP in the tissue sample increases the sensitivity of the system regardless of whether a univalent or multivalent ^{125}I marker is used. Whether a still greater increase in sensitivity could be achieved by preparing a marker in which iodotyrosine residue is attached to cAMP at some point other than the 2'-OH residue, decreasing the affinity of the marker for antibody but increasing the ability of unlabeled 2'O-succinyl cAMP in the sample to compete, is not presently known. Judging from the success in obtaining a satisfactory immunoassay for human prolactin by using an antiserum to ovine prolactin and a porcine prolactin (but not an ovine prolactin) marker (see above), it may not always be desirable to make the marker as much like the hapten on the immunizing conjugate as possible, since doing so may create a situation in which the binding of the marker is greatly favored.

ANTIBODY HETEROGENEITY

The Mathematical Expression of Heterogeneity

As another means of expressing binding between an antibody and a hapten, equation (1) can be reexpressed as

$$(3) \qquad\qquad K_a \;=\; \frac{r}{(n-r)c}$$

where r is the molar concentration of bound antibody sites at equilibrium [not the gas constant as used in equation (2) of Chapter 2], c is the molar concentration of free hapten, n is the molar concentration of total antibody sites, and $n - r$ is the molar concentration of free antibody sites. The graphic presentation of equation (2) plotting r/c versus r is known as a Scatchard plot. It was first applied to the study of antibody binding by Eisen and Karush (1949). When a wide range of hapten concentration is covered the plot can be used to determine the total number of antibody combining sites (n) as calculated from the extrapolated intercept on the abscissa; the slope is $-K_a$. A typical Scatchard plot for the binding of Lac hapten by anti-Lac antibody is presented in Fig. 6.2. It will be noted that the plot of Lac binding is not a straight line. This is a reflection of differences of hapten binding between different subpopulations of antibody. Such antibody heterogeneity is a complicating factor in quantitative studies of binding affinity. In haptenic systems, however, binding can usually be adequately approximated by the introduction of a heterogeneity index into

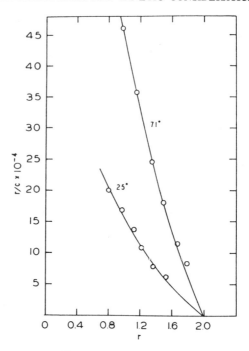

Fig. 6.2. Binding results at 25° and 7.1° C for the reaction between Lac dye and purified anti-Lac antibody. The points are experimental and the curves are theoretical. (Taken from F. Karush. 1957. J. Am. Chem. Soc. 79:3380-3384.)

the binding equation. The most satisfactory mathematical treatment for heterogeneity involves the use of a Sipsian function (Nisonoff and Pressman, 1958; Karush, 1962)

$$(4) \qquad \log \frac{r}{n-r} = a \log C + a \log K_{\bar{a}}$$

where K_a is the average association constant and a is given by the slope in a plot of $\log (r/n - r)$ versus $\log C$. The equation is obtained by rearrangement of equation (3) and reduction to logarithms (Nisonoff and Pressman, 1958; Karush, 1962). If the antibody is homogeneous, a plot of $\log (r/n - r)$ versus $\log C$ will yield a straight line with a regression coefficient (slope) of 1.0 ($a = 1$). If the antibody is not homogeneous but there is a normal distribution of antibody affinities in the sample, the plot will continue to take a straight line, with the magnitude of the heterogeneity being reflected in the degree of deviation of a from 1.0, where 0 represents maximal heterogeneity. Under these conditions the average affinity K_0 can easily be estimated from the K_a when one-half the antibody sites are occupied. At the point, $r = n - r$, and equation (4) becomes

(5) $$a \log C + a \log K_0 = 0$$

(6) $$a \log K_0 = -a \log C$$

(7) $$K_0 = 1/C$$

Thus K_0, the average binding constant, is given by the concentration of C at which one-half the antibody sites are occupied.

Studies of Antibody Heterogeneity by
Direct Binding Measurements

As a rule, equation (4) appears to be an adequate approximation of antibody binding. However, the studies of Werblin and Siskind (1972) with anti-DNP antibodies obtained at different times after immunization indicate that such is not always the case, as indicated by nonlinearity particularly in the late stages of immunization. Late antisera tend to have in a plot of log $(r/n - r)$ versus log C with some antibody preparations, two major populations of antibodies, one of low affinity and one of high affinity, and at present there is no satisfactory means of expressing the binding heterogeneities of such antisera mathematically. Despite these exceptions, a is a valuable quantitative index of antibody heterogenity. Most antibody preparations exhibit considerable binding heterogeneity with values of a ranging from 0.3 to 0.8 (when a is 0.5, 20% of the sites in the sample of antibody molecules have K values that fall outside the range between $K_0/40$ and $40/K_0$). Thus a low value for a means a broad spread of antibody affinities but not necessarily an unusually large number of antibody species. Occasionally homogeneous binding with a value for a of 1.0 is reported; but in most such studies binding has not been evaluated over a several log range of hapten concentrations, and it is possible that some low-affinity antibody is being missed.

Antibody Fractionation

In addition to direct binding studies, antibody heterogeneity can be demonstrated by fractional precipitation (or absorption) in which small amounts of antigen are successively added to an antiserum and the bound antibody is isolated and purified after each addition. The initial fractions contain the antibody of highest affinity with a progressive fall in affinity as later fractions are examined. The question arises as to whether, for radioimmunoassay purposes, there is merit in fractionating antibodies so that high-affinity antibodies can be utilized as a relatively pure population. The answer depends largely on whether the antibody or the antigen is being labeled. In an immunoassay utilizing a radioiodinated antibody marker, purification is often desirable for maximal sensitivity (because of the importance of keeping binding by "nonspecific" gamma globulin to insolubilized antigen to a minimum). In assays involving labeled antigens, specific purification of antibody generally is unnecessary and may be undesirable because of possible losses of high-affinity antibody during purification. Consider, for example, the problems involved in the purification of anti-DNP antibody. One method of purification is to absorb the antibody to a DNP-containing resin. Once the antibody has been absorbed, it must be recovered from the resin, either by the addition of hapten or by a change in pH or ionic strength. However, unless conditions that lead to partial antibody denaturation are used, antibody recovery is always less than 100%. In immunoassay applications, this loss of antibody is of special concern, since it is the high-affinity antibody that is especially difficult to recover. Moreover, when hapten elution procedures are used, the hapten is often difficult to remove, and any antibody molecules that retain the hapten (again, primarily the segment with highest affinity) will be blocked as far as combining with marker is concerned. Another reason why most immunoassays do not utilize specifically purified antibodies is that under the usual assay conditions low-affinity antibodies do not participate to an important extent in binding. With heterogeneous populations of antibody at dilutions that permit maximal immunoassay sensitivity, it can be assumed that the higher-affinity antibody molecules preferentially bind the hapten. A significant contribution to binding by low-affinity antibodies is likely only after much larger amounts of hapten are added and the high-affinity antibody sites become largely saturated. In essence, the high-affinity antibody sites are titrated first, the low-affinity antibody being largely bypassed. Thus specific purification of antibody would normally not be necessary even if losses of high-affinity antibody during purification were not a problem.

When sera are being evaluated for use in radioimmunoassays, there is no real need to define the entire range of antibody affinities. What is usually done is to dilute the antibody and determine empirically the maximal sensitivity of the system. This process provides an operational estimate of useful affinity even though the average K_a for the antibody population as a whole is not known.

KINETICS OF THE ANTIGEN-ANTIBODY REACTION

Kinetics of Antibody-Hapten Interactions

The reaction between antibody and hapten can be described in kinetic terms by k_1 and k_2, the rate constants for association and dissociation, respectively.

$$(8) \qquad Ab + H \underset{k_2}{\overset{k_1}{\rightleftharpoons}} Ab \cdot H$$

At equilibrium, the association constant K_a is the ratio of k_1/k_2. The forward reaction is so fast that it cannot be measured by conventional binding techniques. A method that lends itself to rate measurements is fluorescence quenching, which is based on the ability of chromphoric haptens to diminish antibody fluorescence (Velick et al., 1960; Parker, et al., 1966). Even at concentrations as low as 40-nmolar anti-DNP antibody and 90-nmolar ε-DNP-lysine, the reaction is largely complete within 64 ms (Day et al., 1963) (Fig. 6.3). Based on these and similar experiments with haptens that undergo spectral shifts following combination with antibody, it is clear that values for k_1 can be very high, in the range of 10^7 to 10^8 liters mole^{-1} s^{-1} (Day et al., 1963; Froese and Sehon, 1965; Froese, 1968). This range approaches the theoretical limit of 10^9 liters mole^{-1} s^{-1} calculated for diffusion-controlled reactions (in this case, a reaction determined by the frequency of collision between hapten and antibody molecules, assuming that the hapten is spherically symmetrical and uncharged). In experiments with anti-DNP antibody, the apparent activation energy is low, in the region of 4 kcal/mole^{-1}. Presumably much or all of this energy is consumed in overcoming solvent viscosity. In view of the high forward association constant and low activation energy, a major configurational change in the antibody during its initial interaction with hapten is unlikely (Day et al., 1963). This conclusion is in agreement with those drawn from sedimentation velocity studies of free antibody and antibody-hapten complexes that fail to distinguish between bound and free antibody (Warner et al., 1970).

Kinetics of Protein-Antiprotein Interactions

Less information is available on the k_1 for protein-antiprotein interactions. In fluorescence polarization studies utilizing fluorescein-labeled

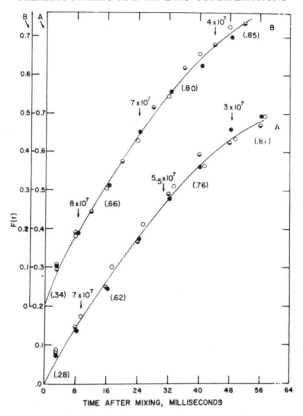

Fig. 6.3. Kinetics of reaction of anti-DNP antibody with (a) DNP lysine and (b) DNP amino-caproate at 25°C, plotted as a second-order forward, first-order reverse reaction. Initial concentration of Ab sites, 4.7 x 10⁻⁷ M; of hapten, 9.4 x 10⁻⁷ M. Closed, open, and shaded circles refer to three separate runs. Numbers in parentheses indicate fraction of total Ab sites reacted at different points on the curves. Included above the curves are apparent second-order rate constants calculated from tangents at various points indicated by the arrows. (Taken from L. A. Day, J. M. Sturtevant, and S. J. Singer. 1963. Ann. N.Y. Acad. Sci. 103:611-625.)

protein antigens, a value of 2×10^5 mole^{-1} has been obtained for the ovalbumin-antiovalbumin system, suggesting that k_1 may be considerably lower for proteins than for haptens. This premise is not surprising, since proteins diffuse less rapidly and have a more elaborate three-dimensional structure (with the possibility of steric hindrance or problems in properly aligning the antibody and antigen), areas that are inactive immunologically, and determinants that might conceivably need to undergo a conformational change when they interact with antibody. Thus there is a much greater possibility of an ineffective collision in the case of a protein than of a hapten. At very low concentrations of antigen and antibody, the low k_1

would tend to delay equilibration and explain in part the greater time required for sensitive immunoassay measurements in protein than in haptenic systems.

Kinetic measurements also provide an interesting insight into the difference in binding properties of high-and low-affinity antibodies. Values of k_1 for high-affinity anti-DNP antibodies ($K \sim 1 \times 10^8$ liters mole^{-1}) and low-affinity antibenzenearsonate antibodies ($K \sim 1 \times 10^5$ liters mole^{-1}) are surprisingly similar, indicating that the differences in K_a are primarily due to variation in k_2 rather than k_1 (Froese, 1968). In these two systems the calculated values for k_2 are at least fiftyfold lower for high-than for low-affinity antihapten antibodies (1 s^{-1} versus 50 s^{-1}).

Although the rate of association is markedly reduced in protein-antiprotein systems, the rate of dissociation is also reduced. In the ovalburin-antiovalbumin reaction alluded to above, the rate of dissociation was very low (a k_2 of only 1×10^{-3} s^{-1}), which, combined with a k_1 of 2×10^5 mole s^{-1}, gives a calculated K_a of 2×10^8 liters mole^{-1}, which is comparable to that seen in high-affinity DNP/anti-DNP interactions. As already discussed, the opportunity for multivalent interactions undoubtedly contributes to the low k_2 for proteins.

Kinetic Considerations in the Performance of Immunoassays

Information on the kinetics of antibody binding to antigen can be used in attempting to rationalize what happens during the performance of a radioimmunoassay. Since the complexing of hapten to antibody is a bimolecular reaction, it is determined by the product of the absolute concentrations of antigen and antibody [equation (6-1)]. With assays conducted at very low concentrations of reactants, equilibration will be delayed. In the foregoing example involving the reaction of 40-nmolar anti-DNP antibody with 90-nmolar ϵ-DNP-lysine, the reaction was essentially complete within 0.1 s, but if the concentrations of the two reactants had each been reduced a hundredfold, equilibration would have taken at least 10,000 times as long (16 minutes). The time required would actually be longer than 16 minutes, since the longer association time would provide a greater opportunity for dissociation during the initial forward reaction. A curve for differences in cAMP marker binding to anti-cAMP antibody with time is shown in Fig. 6.4. It is apparent that binding is not maximal until many hours have elapsed. Extrapolating to protein-antiprotein systems where the k_1 is much lower and reactant concentrations are frequently in the picomolar range, it is not hard to understand why at least several days may be needed in order to obtain maximal assay sensitivity. Additional factors in the long equilibration time for proteins are the complexity of the antigen-

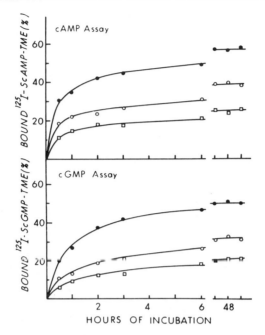

Fig. 6.4. Rate of equilibrium for cAMP and cGMP immunoassays. Bound [^{125}I] ScAMP-TME and [^{125}I] ScGMP-TME were precipitated with 60% (NH$_4$)$_2$SO$_4$ after addition of 200 μg of rabbit IgG. •, absence of added cyclic nucleotide; o, 2 pmoles of cAMP, 0.5 pmole of cGMP; □, 5 pmoles of cAMP, 1 pmole of cGMP. Taken from A. L. Steiner, C. W. Parker, and D. M. Kipnis. 1972. J. Biol. Chem. 247:1106-1113.)

antibody reaction and the opportunity for formation of different types of complexes. Intuitively, we would assume that a variety of complexes are formed initially and that complexes of maximal stability are obtained only after the reaction had proceeded over a substantial period of time.

A similar maximization of complex stability by successive approximation is theoretically possible in antibody-hapten interactions. Although hapten systems equilibrate more rapidly than protein systems, as noted in Fig. 6.4, up to 24 hours may be needed for maximal sensitivity. Even though much of this delay represents time needed for the antibody and the hapten to establish effective contact in dilute solution, theoretical estimates for equilibration times based on approximate antibody and hapten concentrations and binding constants sometimes lead to different (shorter) values than those actually observed. The explanation for this phenomenon has not been carefully studied. The similarity in k_1's for antihapten antibodies of differing affinities creates the theoretical likelihood that, when hapten is limiting, it is distributed initially between high-, intermediate-, and low-affinity antibodies. If this situation occurred, and assay tubes were processed after a short incubation period, the low-affinity complexes would tend to dissociate during the separation of antibody bound from free hapten, thus decreasing the concentration of bound marker and increasing the amount of antibody required to provide a given level of marker binding. As the incubation proceeded, the hapten would be gradually redistributed to the high-affinity antibody. The rate of redistribution would depend on the relative concentrations and k_2's of the various antibodies. In unfavorable circumstances the achievement of a true equilibrium might be delayed for many hours, helping explain why greater sensitivity is obtained with prolonged incubation even though the initial interaction between hapten and antibody occurs more rapidly.

EFFECTS OF TEMPERATURE ON THE ANTIGEN-ANTIBODY REACTION

Effects on Binding at Equilibrium

The influence of temperature on the antigen-antibody reaction varies with the antibody and incubation conditions. In general, the K_a increases as the temperature is lowered, and antigen binding is maximal at or near 4°C, provided that equilibrium is reached. The relationship between K_a and temperature can be described mathematically by the equation

$$(9) \qquad \Delta F° = \Delta H° - T \Delta S°$$

where $\Delta H°$ and $\Delta S°$ represent the enthalpy and entropy contributions to binding, respectively, T is the absolute temperature, and $\Delta F°$ is the standard free energy of binding [see equation (3), Chapter 4]. ΔH is usually negative, a reflection of the decreased binding at increased temperature. An example of the effect of temperature on the binding is given in Fig. 6.2. The magnitude of the enthalpy effect varies widely with the antibody, from relative large to essentially negligible values. Negative values are usually observed even in reactions involving hydrophobic haptens, despite the prediction that the stability of hydrophobic bonds should be unchanged or even increased with increases in temperature. As noted, evidently binding forces that diminish with increasing temperature are also involved, resulting in an overall value for ΔH that is negative. Regardless of the nature of the binding forces involved, if the antigen-antibody system under study is substantially affected by temperature and an assay of maximal sensitivity is required, the final hours of the incubation will need to be carried out at reduced temperatures and the same low temperature must be maintained during subsequent processing for counting. This factor will be especially important in haptenic systems because of the relative high k_2 for dissociation.

Effects on Rapidity of Equilibration

The binding of antigen by antibody is normally improved at low temperatures, but only under equilibrium conditions. The approach to equilibrium is slowed because of the decreased frequency of collision between antigen and antibody. For this reason, many immunoassays utilize a preliminary (usually 15 to 60 minutes) incubation at ambient temperature or 37°C, followed by a longer period of incubation at low temperature. In immunoassays involving large molecular weight protein antigens, an initial 60-minute incubation at 37°C may shorten the overall time requirement in the assay by as much as 24 to 48 hours. (The use of incubation temperatures above 37°C is undesirable because of the danger of antibody denaturation.)

COMPETITIVE AND "NONCOMPETITIVE" BINDING ASSAYS

Equilibrium Competitive Binding Assays

THEORETICAL CONSIDERATIONS

The most frequently used radioimmunoassays involve competitive binding between labeled and unlabeled antigen for the same antibody. This situation can be expressed mathematically as

$$(10) \qquad Ag^*{\cdot}Ab \; \leftrightharpoons \; Ag^* + Ab + Ag \; \rightleftharpoons \; Ag{\cdot}Ab$$

where Ag and Ag* are unlabeled and labeled Ag, respectively. If B is the total concentration of bound antigen, then

$$(11) \qquad B = Ag{\cdot}Ab + Ag^*{\cdot}Ab$$

The optimization of assay conditions is usually worked out empirically, but the problem can also be approached from a theoretical point of view from theoretical mathematic treatments of binding. Drawing heavily on earlier presentations by Ekins et al. (1970) and by Yalow and Berson (1970b), Feldman and Rodbard (1971) have discussed the mathematic variables that affect radioimmunoassay sensitivity in some detail. Is it useful to express binding in terms of R* and R, the ratios of bound to free antigen for labeled and unlabeled antigen, respectively. If Ag* and Ag react indistinguishably with antibody, then

$$(12) \qquad R = R^* = \frac{Ag^*{\cdot}Ab}{Ag^*}$$

In a competitive-binding equilibrium radioimmunoassay involving a homogenous antibody and antigen, the character of the binding curve and the sensitivity of the system for unlabeled Ag depend on three major factors: (a) Ab, the total concentration of antibody, (b) K_a, the association constant of the antibody, and (c) Ag*, the total concentration of labeled antigen. The mathematical relationship between these variables and Ag, the total concentration of unlabeled Ag, is given by

(13) $R^2 + R (1 + K \cdot Ag + K \cdot Ag^* - K \cdot Ab) - K \cdot Ab = 0$

obtained by combining equations (10), (11), and (12). The three variables are interdependent, and the most satisfactory assay system will involve an optimal combination of the three. Equation (13) can be used to construct a theoretical plot to elucidate the effect of varying the antibody concentration when Ag* is very small and K is arbitrarily fixed at 10×10^6 liters /mole. Such a plot is shown in Fig. 6.5. The ordinate is bound/total Ag*. It will be noted that when the smallest amount of Ab is used, the most sensitive curve in terms of inhibition of Ag* binding by unlabeled Ag is obtained. However, the level of Ag* binding when inhibition is absent is only 20%, and the range of unlabeled Ag concentrations

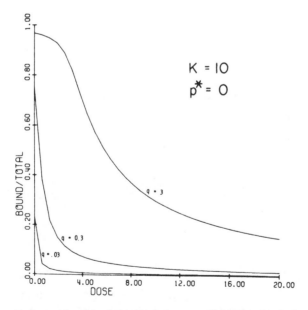

Fig. 6.5. Theoretical curve for the relationship between q, the total concentration of antibody, and inhibition of marker binding by unlabeled antigen when K is arbitrarily fixed at 10×10^6 liters mole^{-1} and the quantity of labeled marker, p*, is infinitely small. (Taken from H. Feldman, and D. Rodbard. 1971. *In* W. D. Odell and W. H. Daughaday (Eds.). Principles of competitive protein-binding assays. J. B. Lippincott Co., Philadelphia. pp. 158-199.)

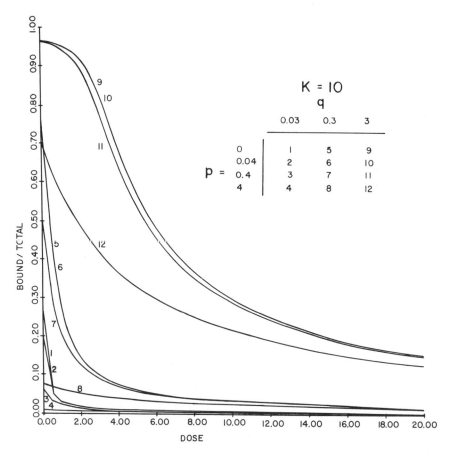

Fig. 6.6. Theoretical curve for the relationship between binding of marker and unlabeled antigen dose when both the total concentration of antibody, q, and the total concentration of marker, p*, are varied. Curves 1 to 4 and 8 have a low starting value because of too little antibody or too much tracer. Curves 9 to 11 have a high starting value as a result of high antibody concentration (q = 3). (Taken from H. Feldman, and D. Rodbard. 1971. *In* W. D. Odell, and W. H. Daughaday (Eds.). *Principles of competitive protein-binding assays.* J. B. Lippincott Co., Philadelphia. pp. 158-199.)

over which inhibition can be followed is limited. The intermediate concentration of antibody represents a compromise between adequate sensitivity and useful levels of Ag* binding. When both Ag* and Ab are varied and *K* is again fixed, another series of curves is obtained (Fig. 6.6). The most sensitive curves are those with very small amounts of Ag* and Ab (curves 1 and 2). However, again the curve is limited in its range, with the amount of radioactivity bound to Ab rapidly becoming vanishingly small.

In this situation, long counting times would be required to obtain statistically valid data. A good compromise between having substantial amounts of bound radioactivity and useful sensitivity is given by curve 7. In curve 7, Ag* is $4/K$, whereas Ab is $3/K$. This is the theoretical relationship between K_1, Ag*, and Ab, suggested by Ekins (1968) as providing the least detectable dose of unlabeled antigen. The assumptions involved in Ekin's derivation are given in the figure legend. One important assumption is that antigen binding by antibody is homogeneous, which it rarely is. Ekin's calculation is made for a B/T ratio of 0.5. Berson and Yalow have suggested that if the calculation is made for very low concentrations of Ag*, a B/T ratio of 0.33 provides the most sensitive curve. As already emphasized, regardless of whether optimal Ag* and antibody concentrations are used, a sensitive inhibition curve is obtained only if the antibody has a high K_a. The effect of K_a on assay sensitivity in the idealized binding system (very small concentrations of Ag* and a total antibody concentration of $3/K$) is illustrated in Fig. 6.7.

It should be pointed out that the preceding discussion is directed toward immunoassay applications in which sensitivity must be maximized. If low levels of sensitivity are needed, the use of generous quantities of reagents will help reduce assay variability. It will also permit the assay to be completed more rapidly.

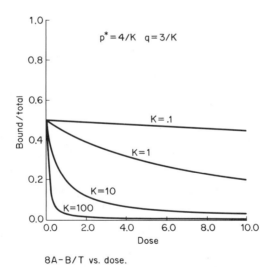

8A−B/T vs. dose.

Fig. 6.7. Theoretical curve for relationship between marker binding and unlabeled antigen dose with antibodies of affinities ranging between 1×10^5 and 1×10^8 liters $mole^{-1}$ when optimal concentrations of marker and antibody are used. (Taken from H. Feldman, and D. Rodbard. 1971. *In* W. D. Odell, and W. H. Daughaday (Eds.). Principles of competitive protein-binding assays. J. B. Lippincott Co., Philadelphia. pp. 158-199.)

In practice, the antibody is rarely homogenous, its average affinity and absolute concentration in serum are not known, and sufficient levels of bound Ag* are needed in order to avoid unduly long counting times. Moreover, in hapten immunoassays, the Ag* and the unlabeled Ag are frequently not equivalent in their binding affinities for antibody. Therefore as Ekins (1974) himself emphasizes, the formulas presented at best provide no more than a rough rule of thumb, and optimal assay conditions must be worked out empirically (see Chapter 7). Where high levels of sensitivity are needed, the procedure followed in our laboratory is to take Ag* at the highest practical specific activity (the maximal labeling level obtainable without significant losses of immunological reactivity), place 8,000 to 15,000 cpm in assay tubes, and determine the minimal concentration of antibody needed to give 30 to 50% binding of the marker. The result gives the minimal concentrations of Ag* and antibody needed to provide practical levels of antibody-bound radioactivity. Ag*, Ab, and the functional K for that concentration of antibody are now fixed, although possibly not at levels that are optimal according to Ekin's criteria.

Nonequilibrium Competitive Binding Assays

Because reequilibration takes place slowly, when high-affinity antibody is involved, there is a theoretical advantage to exposing the antibody to unlabeled Ag—waiting long enough to achieve optimal binding—and then adding Ag* (Fig. 6.8). This procedure gives the unlabeled Ag access to antibody at a time when no Ag* is present, thus increasing its ability to compete. If the time period after the addition of Ag* is limited, a portion of the original advantage will be retained, and a given quantity of Ag will have an exaggerated effect on Ag* binding. Feldman and Rodbard (1971) have calculated theoretical curves for differences in assay sensitivity, depending on whether the Ag or the Ag* is added first. Many laboratories add the inhibitor before the marker, but the final incubation step is sufficiently prolonged (for 16 to 48 hours) that considerable reequilibration is possible, thus reducing the effect of the preincubation. Nonetheless, if the antigen-antibody complexes dissociate slowly, some gain in sensitivity may be retained even in prolonged incubations. Utiger (1974) has found that immunoassay sensitivity for human thyrotropin is increased twofold when the addition of the marker is delayed until the second day even though the total duration of the assay is 5 days. Shorter final incubation periods in the range of 1 to 6 hours can be used, but Ag* binding may

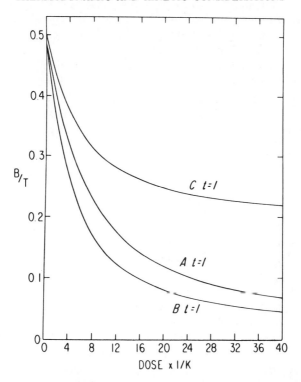

Fig. 6.8. Theoretical curves for relationship between marker binding and unlabeled antigen dose when three different addition sequences are used: Curve A: simultaneous addition of tracer, unlabeled antigen, and antibody. Curve B: delayed addition of tracer, resulting in improved sensitivity and precision. Curve C: delayed addition of unlabeled antigen, resulting in loss of sensitivity and precision. Response was measured one time unit after addition of last reagent. K is arbitrary; $p^* = 4/K$ and $q = 3/K$. (Taken from H. Feldman, and K. Rodbard. 1971. *In* W. D. Odell, and W. H. Daughaday (Eds.). Principles of competitive protein-binding assays. J. B. Lippincott Co., Philadelphia. pp. 158-199.)

be suboptimal in uninhibited controls. Moreover, in assays involving many tubes, if a short final incubation time is used, particular care is needed to minimize intra-assay variations in the duration of the second incubation period or in the manner in which the immunological reagents are mixed. This factor is particularly important in solid-phase systems. Thus the theoretical increase in sensitivity of a nonequilibrium system may not be realized because of reduced Ag* binding and increased assay variability. However, if the sensitivity needed cannot be obtained by other methods, a nonequilibrium system with a relatively brief final incubation may be considered. The degree of success will depend on the method used for incubating and separating the immune reactants and on the range of forward and background kinetic constants for binding in the particular antigen-antibody system under study. Since the use of a nonequilibrium assay may limit Ag* binding by antibody to a smaller percentage of total Ag* than is normally the case, Wide et al. (1973) advocate the use of much higher levels of Ag* radioactivity than are used in equilibrium assays. Such use permits the development of substantial levels of bound antigen radio-activity even though the fraction of the total tracer bound is 10% or less. Obviously a system of this kind requires the rigorous separation of bound antibody from free antigen in order to eliminate large unbound antigen blanks.

"Noncompetitive" Binding Assays

As discussed in Chapter 5, Miles and Hales (1968) have pointed out several disadvantages of conventional competitive binding radioimmuno-assays: (a) Because of the adverse effect of excessive amounts of antibody on assay sensitivity, the investigator may be forced to select conditions in which much of the antigen is not bound to antibody. (b) With some antigens, the preparation of a stable, high-specific activity marker presents major difficulties. (c) There may be antibody subpopulations that bind with greater affinity to the unlabeled than to the labeled antigen. To eliminate some of these disadvantages, Miles and Hales proposed an ingenious two-step "noncompetitive" binding system in which the anti-body rather than the antigen is radioiodinated. In the first step the un-known antigen (bovine insulin) was reacted with excess ^{125}I antibody in solution. In the second step the mixture was exposed to excess insolubilized antigen (unlabeled). In the absence of unknown Ag, the ^{125}I antibody was quantitatively absorbed by the insolubilized antigen (Fig. 6.9). In the presence of insolubilized Ag, the absorption of ^{125}I antibody was partially inhibited, thus providing a quantitative measure of the amount of unknown antigen in the system. Since step I is carried out in ^{125}I antibody excess and step II in insoluble antigen excess, theoretically both reactions proceed stoichiometrically, and there is no competition between unknown antigen and insoluble antigen for antibody. Miles and Hales therefore use the term *noncompetitive immunoassay* to describe the procedure.

How noncompetitive, iodinated antibody immunoassays compare with conventional iodinated antigen assays in terms of sensitivity, precision, and specificity remains to be established conclusively. Oddly enough, ap-parantly there was no direct experimental analysis of the relative sensitivity of labeled antibody and labeled antigen immunoassays (using the same antiserum). Rodbard and Weiss (1973) have discussed the theoretical sensitivity of the two systems and suggested that, because multiple iodines can be introduced onto antibody molecules, the labeled antibody method

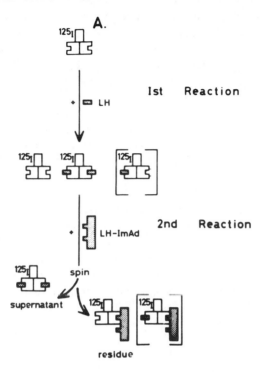

Fig. 6.9. Assay of human luteinizing hormone (LH) using purified radioactive antibodies to human chorionic gonadotropin (^{125}I-anti-HCG-IgG). LH-ImAd $=$ immunoabsorbent-containing luteinizing hormone. The second-site reaction, which would allow antibody already bound to one antigen molecule to bind also to the ImAd, reducing the sensitivity of the assay, is shown in brackets. (Taken from L. E. M. Miles. 1971. *In* W. D. Odell, and W. H. Daughaday (Eds.). Principles of competitive protein-binding assays. J. B. Lippincott Co., Philadelphia. pp. 260-281.)

is theoretically more sensitive. However, no conclusions are possible until a direct experimental comparison of the two methods has been made with identical antisera in several antigen-antibody systems.

Even if additional data seem to favor the use of iodinated antibody immunoassays, several inherent disadvantages to the iodinated antibody approach should be kept in mind:

1. Iodinated antibodies adhere nonspecifically to glassware and insoluble resins just as iodinated antigens do; and since the iodinated antibody is used in excess, the problem may be magnified. For this reason, the method used for insolubilizing the antigen is critical in maintaining nonspecific binding at an acceptable level. Although insolubilized antigens with relatively little nonspecific affinity for iodinated immunoglobulins have been prepared in a number of antigen-antibody systems, it is not certain that it will always be possible to do so, and extensive preliminary

investigation may be needed. Nonspecific binding can be considerably diminished by preparing Fab fragments of the labeled antibody, but this procedure might reduce the avidity of the antibody for antigen on the resin and adversely affect assay sensitivity. In studies of bacteriophage inactivation referred to earlier, Hornick and Karush (1969) found a one hundredfold reduction in the functional avidity of anti-DNP antibody for DNP phage after reduction to Fab fragments, and this finding is further illustrated by studies with anti-red-cell antibodies (Fig. 6.10).

2. Substantial amounts of unlabeled antigen are needed to prepare the resin, which may preclude the use of this approach for antigens that are in short supply.

3. Specifically purified antibodies, ideally, should be used for iodination and binding in order to optimize sensitivity and specificity. In some antigen-antibody systems major difficulties are encountered in obtaining satisfactory preparations of purified antibody. Thus the system is more wasteful both of antigen and of antibody.

4. Since only a relatively small proportion of the iodinated antibody is complexed to antigen and excess insoluble antigen is used during the second phase of the reaction, problems may arise in antigen-antibody

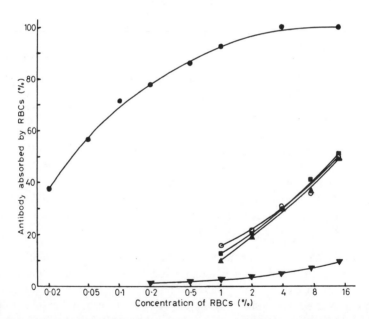

Fig. 6.10. Avidity of bivalent and univalent 5S and 3.5S anti-A antibodies for human red cells containing A antigen. (●) Bivalent 5S; univalent 5S; (■) 3.5S (reduced 5S that did not recombine); (▲) 3.5S (reduced alkylated 5S). Red cells of type O (▼) were used to measure nonspecific uptake. (Taken from C. L. Greenbury, D. H. Moore, and L. A. C. Nunn. 1965. Immunology, 8:420-431.)

systems in which the rate of dissociation of antigen from antibody is relatively rapid [a high k_2; see equation (8)]. Although theoretically the system is noncompetitive, in practice, during phase II signification dissociation and reequilibration of immune complexes are likely to take place unless an immune system with unusually stable antigen complexes is involved. Thus the kinetics of dissociation of the antigen-antibody complex may have a marked effect on the sensitivity of the system, just as is true in nonequilibrium, competitive binding systems, and this approach is more likely to be useful in immunoassays for proteins than for haptens. Even in protein systems the iodination reaction must be controlled so as to avoid excess iodination of the antibody. Otherwise the antibody may dissociate too rapidly from the resin (Fig. 6.11).

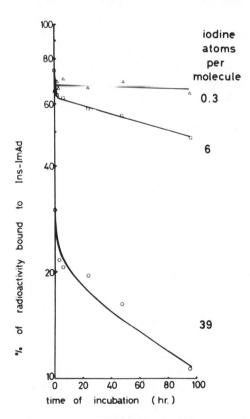

Fig. 6.11. Rate of dissociation of trace-labeled ^{125}I-antiinsulin antibody from its complex with insulin immunoabsorbent (insulin-ImAd). Preparations containing 0.3, 6, and 39 atoms of [127]I per molecule of IgG were reacted with insulin-ImAd. When equilibrium was reached, excess soluble insulin was added (at time = 0), and the fall in ImAd-bound radioactivity with time was followed. (Taken from L. E. M. Miles. 1971. *In* W. D. Odell, and W. H. Daughaday. (Eds.). Principles of competitive protein-binding assays. J. B. Lippincott Co., Philadelphia. pp. 260-281.)

QUANTITATION OF ANTIBODY BY RADIOIMMUNOASSAY

Antibodies as well as antigens can be measured by radioimmunoassay methods. One commonly used approach is to prepare multiple dilutions of the antiserum and measure radioactive antigen binding with each. As described originally by Farr (1958, 1971), if the antigen is soluble in 40 or 50% ammonium sulfate, free and bound antigen can easily be separated and the antigen-binding activity of a serum determined. The titer of a serum is ordinarily expressed as the reciprocal of the highest dilution giving an arbitrary level of antigen binding (usually 33%). However, because of the normal heterogeneity of antibodies in regard to binding affinity, binding in relatively dilute antigen-antibody solutions is a function both of antibody concentration and of affinity. If low-affinity antibody is present, only a portion of the antibody is detected. This uncertainty is partially rectified by carrying out binding measurements at several levels of antigen, but even then precise quantitation is not obtained. Osler (1971) has suggested a simple modification of the Farr assay that provides an accurate measure of the antibody content of a serum even in highly diluted samples. The essential feature is that a very broad range of antigen concentrations is covered while keeping the level of antibody constant. This process provides information on antigen binding when marked excesses of antigen are present. Assuming that much or all of the antibody is utilized for binding under these conditions, that IgG antibodies are involved, and that most or all of the complexes have an Ag_2Ab configuration, the maximal level of bound antigen can be used to calculate the total quantity of antibody present. Calibration curves in which immune sera containing known amounts of precipitating antibody were diluted and measured for maximal antigen-binding capacity in this system have given highly satisfactory results in terms of antibody recovery, thereby indicating the general validity of the preceding assumptions. It should be noted, however, that because of the large excesses of radiolabeled antigen used, this approach requires that a very clean separation of bound from free antigen be obtainable.

As discussed above and in Chapter 5, another approach to the measurement of small quantities of antibody is to incubate a solid-phase immunoabsorbant containing the antigen with the unknown antiserum. The absorbant is washed and bound antibody is determined by means of a radiolabeled second antibody. If class-specific second antibodies are used, this procedure is applicable to measurement of antibodies in individual immunoglobulin classes. However, it is also susceptible to variations in antibody affinity.

Summary

1. Factors influencing the sensitivity of immunoassays include the equilibrium constant for the antibody-antigen reaction, the rate of dissociation of complexes during separation of free and bound antigen, incubation conditions, antigen and antigen body valence, and the relative immunological reactivities of labeled and unlabeled antigen.

2. Association (K_a) or avidity (K_{avid}) constants for antibody-hapten and antibody-protein interactions range between 1×10^4 and 1×10^{13} liters /mole^{-1}. The practical sensitivity of an immunoassay is approximately equal to $1/K_a$ or $1/K_{avid}$.

3. As a rule, antisera contain a mixture of antibodies that differ considerably in their affinity for antigen. In general, however, there is no need to fractionate the antiserum, since in the highly diluted solutions of antigen and antibody used in sensitive immunoassays, the low-affinity antibodies do not participate extensively in binding.

4. The stability of antigen-antibody complexes is increased when both the antigen and the antibody are multivalent, thus leading to lattice formation. This is an important factor in the high sensitivity of immunoassays for protein antigens and is reflected by a high K_{av} (the overall avidity of antibody for antigen).

5. In haptenic systems structural differences between the marker and the unlabeled hapten can have an important effect on assay sensitivity. The use of a multivalent hapten marker helps stabilize the marker-anti-hapten-antibody complex, but this step may be self-defeating because the ability of unlabeled hapten to compete with the marker is reduced. Under favorable circumstances hapten present in tissue samples can be chemically altered in situ, increasing its structural resemblance to the form of the hapten on the immunizing antigen and rendering it better able to compete in the immunoassay.

6. The need to identify optimal incubation conditions depends on the characteristics and sensitivity requirements of the immune system in question. When maximal sensitivity is needed, it is necessary to select the antiserum used with care, to minimize the quantity of antibody and radio-labeled antigens used in the assay, and to preincubate the antibody with unknown, unlabeled antigen for an extended period prior to the condition of marker. Long incubation times are more helpful in increasing assay sensitivity in protein than in hapten immunoassays. Preincubation of the unlabeled antigen with antibody renders it better able to compete with antibody, particularly if the incubation is not unduly prolonged once the marker has been added to the system (e.g., if the assay is performed

under nonequilibrium conditions). The potential gain in sensitivity using nonequilibrium conditions is greater with protein than with hapten immunoassays because of the lower rate of dissociation of preformed antigenantibody complexes. If nonspecific binding is not a major problem, it may be advantageous to utilize an unusually large quantity of labeled antigen and introduce it only a few minutes before the reaction is terminated.

7. Attempts to maximize sensitivity may be associated with increased assay variability or susceptibility to nonspecific interference from substances present in tissue. Where a comfortable margin of sensitivity is available, it may be possible to use higher concentrations of antibody and marker and complete the assay much more rapidly, frequently in less than an hour. The assay conditions that lead to maximal sensitivity vary considerably with the immune system, the species immunized, and even the individual antiserum. Nonetheless, if experience with the immune system in other laboratories exists, it will usually provide a useful first approximation in efforts to optimize the assay.

8. The use of an immunoassay system in which the antibody rather than the antigen is labeled presents certain theoretical advantages. The antibody is tagged with ^{125}I, is preincubated with tissue extract antigen (in antibody excess), and is then absorbed to insolubilized antigen (in insolubilized antigen excess). Since there is no direct competition between the unknown tissue antigen and the solid-phase antigen, the term "noncompetitive" has been used to describe the system. However, because the assay is carried out in insolubilized antigen excess, competition obviously can and will occur if the time of exposure of ^{125}I antibody to insolubilized antigen is unduly prolonged or if the stability of preformed complexes between tissue antigen and antibody is not high. Thus this system is critically dependent on the kinetic dissociation constant, k_2, for the antigen-antibody complex in question. In addition, an insolubilized antigen preparation that binds to the iodinated antibody with a high degree of specificity is needed.

9. Antibodies as well as antigens can be quantitated by radioimmunoassay. One approach is to use a solid-phase antigen; binding of antibody to the solid phase is measured by using a radiolabeled second antibody. Another approach is to use a conventional immune precipitation system in which radiolabeled antigen binding is measured. If a broad range of radioactive antigen concentrations is covered, an accurate estimate of the total antibody concentration can be obtained.

Chapter 7

Antiserum Selection and the Mechanics
of the Immunoassay

Selection of Antisera

As discussed elsewhere, careful screening of antisera is important in optimizing the immunoassay. One approach is to incubate a wide range of dilutions of antibody with radioiodinated antigen for 1 to 2 days and determine binding—in effect, utilizing the radiommunoassay itself to select sera. Macroscopic immunoprecipitin techniques, although limited in sensitivity, can also be useful for initial antiserum screening, especially if radio-labeled antigen of established purity is not available. Agar gel diffusion and immunoelectrophoresis are of particular value in that they are simple to perform and provide information both on immunological cross-reactivity and on the presence or absence of multiple antigen-antibody systems. However, if a pure radioactive antigen is available, these analyses are just as easily made in the radioimmunoassay itself. Difficulties can arise when macroscopic precipitation methods are used to screen for antihapten antibodies. Unless a coprecipitating system is used or the hapten is multi-valent, precipitation does not occur. But if the original immunizing hapten-protein conjugate is used to obtain precipitation, some of the precipitation may be due to to antiprotein or anticoupling agent antibodies. Problems in interpretation can be avoided by using a different protein carrier and coupling agent or by demonstrating that precipitation is indeed inhibited when univalent hapten is present. In addition, nonspecific or ineffective precipitation of hapten-protein conjugates may occur because of extensive antigen cross linking or low haptenic substitution. Neutralization of the biological activity of the antigen is another form of screening that can be attempted, although in some antigen-antibody systems a failure to observe inactivation does not exclude the presence of high-affinity antibodies.

Once antisera with intermediate or high titers have been identified, they are evaluated further for maximal sensitivity, steepness, linearity, and reproducibility of standard inhibition curves, cross-reactivity, and susceptibility to nonspecific inhibition in tissue samples and buffer (see below), and those that appear to fulfill the overall requirements of the immunoassay best are selected.

REACTION VOLUMES AND DILUENT SOLUTIONS

As a rule, assays are conducted in a final volume of 0.25 to 0.5 ml. Suitable buffers for dilution include phosphate, borate, or trisbuffered saline. However, ideally, a careful examination of the effect of buffer, pH, ionic strength, and divalent cations should always be made in order to maximize sensitivity and anticipate unexpected sources of interference in the assay. Although assays are usually carried out at neutrality, doing so is not always optimal. In the original cAMP immunoassay, the sensitivity of the system was found to be markedly affected by ionic strength and pH (Steiner et al., 1969; Steiner et al., 1972). Up to tenfold greater sensitivity was obtained in 0.05 M acetate, pH 5.5 to 6.2, than in solutions buffered in the 7.4 to 8.5-pH range. The combined effect of ionic strength and buffer pH would suggest that an electrostatic interaction between the antibody and the hapten is being affected, with an unfavorable effect on the ionization of at least one interacting group as the pH is raised. Interestingly, however, the effect of pH was discovered empirically and would not necessarily have been predicted (the C-6 amino group of cAMP has a pK_a of about 4.2, whereas the pK_a for the basic dissociation on the adenine ring is above 9). It is possible that there is altered ionization of one of these two groups on cAMP when it is sequestered in the antibody-combining site, helping explain the change in binding with pH (Steiner et al., 1972).

Buffer pH may also affect immunoassay specificity. In a recently described immunoassay for human parathyroid hormone (PTH) (Fischer et al., 1974), in which the analytic reagents are anti-PTH fragment (1–12) antibody and a ^{125}I-intact PTH (1–84) marker, the inhibitory capacities of fragment (1–12), fragment (1–34), and intact PTH (1–84) were compared at pH 5 and pH 8.6. The relative inhibitory capacity of PTH (1–12) was increased severalfold at pH 5. Evidently PTH (1–84) and PTH (1–34) both undergo a conformational change as the solution is made more acid, rendering them less able to compete in the immunoassay.

Nonspecific adherence of antigens and haptens (especially hydrophobic haptens) to glass and plastic tubes or pipets may markedly influence measured activity in the immunoassay. With some proteins and polypeptides (ACTH and parthormone, for example), nonspecific binding is reduced if plastic tubes are used. Adherence of hydrophobic haptens can be minimized both by the use of plastic vessels and pipets and by the incorporation of low (1 to 3%, vol: vol) concentrations of methanol, dimethylsulfoxide, or ethanol into hapten-containing solutions or even the final assay mixture. However, too high a concentration of organic solvent in the immunoassay may interfere with the antibody-hapten interaction. Assays involving iodinated antigens are generally carried out in protein-containing buffers. (This procedure is less likely to be desirable in hapten assays.) Bovine serum albumin, gelatin, lysozyme, and ovalbumin are commonly used, usually at final concentrations of 1 to 5 mg/ml. In some systems diluted whole serum or proteins present in the sample itself are just as satisfactory. The addition of protein to the medium minimizes non-specific absorption of the marker and also helps avoid denaturation of highly diluted antigens and antibodies. However, even though added proteins are often beneficial, they should not be used indiscriminately. Albumins, for example, may interfere to some extent in assays involving hydrophobic haptens, because of nonspecific binding. And in assays involving labile antigens, the possibility that proteins in the diluent might contain enzymes that degrade the antigen must be considered.

Possible additives, apart from buffer and protein, include enzyme inhibitors and chelating agents. In assays lasting longer than 3 or 4 days, a bacteriostatic agent, such as Na azide, 0.1 to 0.2%, may be incorporated into the medium to help avoid microbial growth.

ASSAY CONDITIONS

In general, antibody, buffer, and nonradioactive antigen are mixed and radioactive antigen is added after some delay, giving the unlabeled antigen an opportunity to bind to the antibody first. Depending on whether an equilibrium or nonequilibruim assay is being used, the radioactive antigen may be added early in the assay or just before the assay is terminated. By and large, the gain in sensitivity by delayed addition of antigen is much greater in protein than in hapten systems. Assay conditions can vary widely with total incubation times extending from a few minutes to as long as 6 days and should be optimized for the immune system in question. An initial relatively short incubation (5 to 60 minutes) at 37°C or room temperature helps accelerate immune complex formation, but almost all assays are completed in the cold. At the completion of the assay, free and bound antigen are separated. (Methods for separating free and bound Ag are discussed in Chapter 8).

ASSAY CONTROLS

As a part of every assay, several calibration or control measurements must be made:

1. Determination of total antigen radioactivity added to the assay.

2. Determination of nonspecific marker binding (counts present when samples containing the antigen marker but no antibody are processed).

3. Possibly, incubation controls for damage to the immunoreactivity of the radioactive antigen when tissue extracts are present (see Chapter 5).

4. Standard antigen inhibition curves in buffer (and sometimes in tissue extracts as well).

5 Extraction blank or pharmacologic stimulator blank controls, especially if special extraction procedures or new reagents are being utilized.

THE ANTISERUM

The average gamma globulin concentration in animal serum is about 10 mg/ml, although this figure is rather variable and may change to some extent following immunization. Even in hyperimmune sera the percentage of the total gamma globulin that is specific for the immunizing antigen is rarely more than 20%, and frequently antibody levels are considerably lower. In the assay, usually the minimal quantity of antibody giving the desired level of radioactive antigen binding is used (generally 30 to 50% of the total radioactive antigen added). Depending on the antibody and the immune system, this may represent an antiserum dilution of anywhere from 1:100 to 1:1,000,000. The adequacy of antigen binding must be verified in tissue extracts under the conditions in which the assay will be used. Where there is a margin of sensitivity in the system assay, reproducibility may be increased by using more antibody and setting the sensitivity of the system at a lower working level. However, in this case, more tissue sample must be used and problems of nonspecific interference or cross-reactivity may increase.

As a rule, the antiserum is used without purification, particularly when high dilutions of antibody are employed. In certain situations purified gamma globulin fractions are used in order to eliminate serum proteins with undesirable enzymatic or nonspecific binding activity. Almost all the binding activity in hyperimmune sera is in the IgG fraction, so conventional purification procedures for IgG, such as ammonium sulfate precipitation or chromatography on DEAE cellulose, can be used. Albumin and most enzymes in serum can be largely eliminated by ammonium sulfate precipitation at 1.6 M ammonium sulfate. If greater purification is needed, the antibody can be purified further by chromatography on DEAE cellulose, at or near neutral pH. Since IgG has only a small, net, negative charge as neutrality, it has little affinity for DEAE cellulose and is eluted in low-ionic-strength buffer (for a representative procedure, see Parker et al., 1967a). Other serum proteins are retained on the resin. The recovery of antibodies to negatively charged or neutral antigens following this procedure is very good, usually 80% or higher. However, some caution is needed with antibodies to positively charged antigens, since antibodies vary to some extent in their overall charge, depending on their specificity, and this factor may affect their behavior on ion exchange resins. Antibodies to positively charged proteins have a relatively high overall negative charge and adhere to DEAE cellulose, which is positively charged, more avidly than most IgG antibodies do (Sela and Mozes, 1966).

As discussed in Chapter 6, specific purification of antibody to eliminate "nonspecific" IgG is normally unnecessary unless the antibody is to be iodinated instead of the antigen. On the other hand, the use of absorption procedures to remove cross-reactivity antibodies can be helpful in improving specificity (see Chapter 11). IgG antibodies can also be degraded to univalent fragments, but this process generally presents no advantages and may be undesirable if the antigen is multivalent, since the functional avidity of reaction may be reduced.

As noted, it is desirable to include a set of blank tubes in each assay, containing radioactive antigen and buffer or naive serum (diluted in the same way as the antiserum). These tubes are processed just as if antibody were present and provide a measure of the nonspecific binding blank. (It should be kept in mind that nonspecific sticking may be different in buffer than it is in tissue or naive serum.)

Antisera ordinarily can be stored at $-20°C$ for at least 3 to 4 years with little or no detectible loss in immunologic reactivity. Storage is preferably done in small volumes so that antisera need not be repeatedly thawed and refrozen. Once antisera have been diluted, some degree of instability should be assumed even in the frozen state, and fresh dilutions should be prepared frequently.

THE TISSUE EXTRACT

Problems in obtaining tissue extracts suitable for assay are discussed in detail in Chapter 9, as is the importance of ensuring that control measurements are made under conditions as much like those present in tissue samples as possible. All or any portion of the tissue sample may be measured. Sample sizes that bring the level of immunoinhibitory activity within the range of the standard curve are chosen. When the level of antigen in a tissue is variable, it may be desirable to divide tissue extracts into several portions and assay small and large aliquots in order to ensure that the inhibitory activity will fall somewhere on the linear part of the standard antigen inhibition curve. Measurements at several sample levels have the added advantage of providing information on whether inhibition curves with endogenous tissue antigens parallel standard antigen inhibition curves in buffer. Such parallelism is a necessary but not sufficient condition for establishing that the inhibitory activity in tissue samples is truly antigen specific. Enzyme-treated or partially purified tissue samples may also be studied as a further means of validating that the assay is detecting, which it should be when tissue samples are measured (see Chapter 9).

If sensitivity is a problem, it is sometimes possible to concentrate antigen in the tissue extract by specific or nonspecific absorption. For example, using insolubilized specific antibody, Weintraub (1970) was able to increase markedly the sensitivity of an immunoassay for human chorionic somatomammotropin (HCS). Sizable volumes of plasma containing HCS or partially purified HCS were passed through columns of Sepharose-coupled antibody to HCS prior to radioimmunoassay (Fig. 7.1). Any HCS absorbed to columns was then eluted with 6 M guanidine. After the

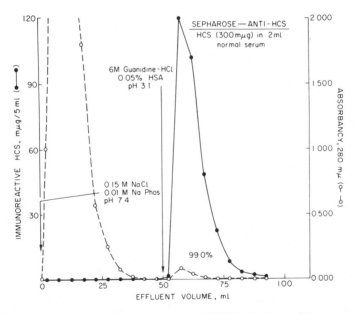

Fig. 7.1. Application of human chorionic somatotropin HCS in 2 ml normal human serum to a column of Sepharose-anti-HCS. No hormone, as measured by radioimmunoassay, appeared in the unretarded fraction, whereas 99% was recovered in the guanidine eluate. Human serum albumin (HSA) was added to the guanidine solution, and it served as a blank in measuring increments of absorbancy in the eluate. The small eluate peak (about 1% applied absorbancy) was not attributable to HCS and represented nonspecific absorption of serum proteins. (Taken from B. D. Weintraub. 1970. Biochem. Biophys. Res. Commun. 39:83-89.)

quanidine had been removed, the sample was concentrated and measured by radioimmunoassay. Up to 500-fold increases in immunoassay sensitivity with apparent recoveries of 85 to 95% were estimated by using this approach. This and similar selective concentration procedures provide a powerful approach to the quantitation of substances too dilute to be measured by routine methods. However, a number of important pitfalls should be kept in mind. They include a failure to obtain quantitative absorption or elution of antigen or inadvertent concentration of cross-reacting or nonspecific interfering substances at the same time that the antigen is concentrated.

THE RADIOACTIVE ANTIGEN

Most assays are carried out at a level of radioactive antigen (in uninhibited samples) of 30 to 50%. Generally bound rather than free radioactivity is determined because the relative change when inhibitor is present is greater. If 8,000 cpm of radioactive antigen is added to the sample and the binding is 30% (in uninhibited samples) the result will provide a maximum of 2,400 cpm of bound radioactivity and a coefficient of variation of about 2% if samples are counted for 1 minute. Although lower levels of total and bound radioactivity can be used, the gain in sensitivity is usually not that great, and the need for longer counting times or the greater statistical variation in counting if 1-minute counts are used is a decided disadvantage. Thus the quantity of radioactive antigen in the assay is fixed by the practical level of bound radioactivity that is required.

Even though radioactive antigen binding is normally maintained in the 30 to 50% range in order to maximize sensitivity, it is important to establish at some point that at least 80 to 90% binding is achievable when larger quantities of antibody are used. This factor provides evidence against major losses in antigenic reactivity as a result of denaturation or iodination. However, it does not necessarily prove the absence of a contaminating antigen-antibody system (see Chapter 9).

THE STANDARD CURVE

A standard curve is included in every assay. It helps provide for the spontaneous variations seen in the assay from day to day. It is also a means of detecting deterioration of the radioactive antigen or an incorrect dilution of antibody. Ideally, incubation mixtures containing standard and unknown antigen should be identical in every respect. If antigen-free tissue samples are not available (and they rarely are), the best approach is to carry out standard curves both in buffer and in tissue extracts. However, this approach is not completely satisfactory, for the standard curve in tissue is superimposed on the background of tissue antigen (see Chapter 9).

The standard curve should cover a broad range of antigen concentrations, extending from minimal to complete inhibition of radioactive antigen binding. While twofold dilutions are normally used in the working part of the standard curve, a narrower dilution span may be desirable, particularly when standard curves are nonlinear. Since dilutions of standard antigen are generally very dilute, the dilutions must be made accurately, since there is no way of directly verifying the antigen concentration once the dilutions have been made. The instability of highly diluted standard solutions can also be a problem, and, as noted, the inclusion of protein in the medium is sometimes desirable so as to minimize denaturation. Obvious problems in interpretation arise when the standard antigen itself is impure or was obtained from a heterologous species.

CALCULATIONS OF TISSUE VALUES

A number of ways of handling the experimental data have been recommended, and there is no general agreement as to what is truly optimal. Examples of different types of graphical analyses are shown in Fig. 7.2. The bias in our laboratory is that the following two procedures are at least as satisfactory as the other methods.

By a Graph of Bound Antigen versus the Log of the Total Unlabeled Antigen Concentration

One simple approach is to plot the standard curve as absolute or percent counts precipitated (ordinate) versus the logarithm of the total unlabeled antigen concentration (abscissa) (Fig. 7.3) and determine the antigen content of tissue samples from where they fall on the standard antigen curve. There is no real advantage in correcting each sample for nonspecific binding, since the blank is already built in to the standard curve. Nor is there any advantage in reexpressing the counts precipitated as ratio of bound to free antigen or even as percent counts bound (although obviously some consideration must be given as to whether the expected level of radioactive antigen binding is being seen). Despite the availability of much more elaborate mathematical models for calculating

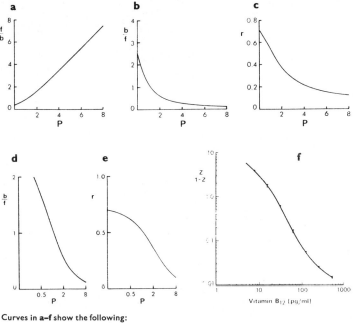

Curves in **a–f** show the following:

a: $\dfrac{\text{free (f)}}{\text{bound (b)}}$ ratio versus ligand concentration

b: $\dfrac{b}{f}$ ratio versus ligand concentration

c: fraction (or percentage) bound (r) versus ligand concentration

d: $\dfrac{b}{f}$ versus log ligand concentration

e: fraction (or percentage) bound (r) versus log ligand concentration

f: logit-type plot $\left(\text{logit } Z = \log \dfrac{Z}{1-Z}, \text{ where } Z = \dfrac{b/f}{b_0/f_0}\right)$; the diagram indicates some, but
   incomplete, linearization of the response curve

It should be noted that the region of maximum slope of the curve depends upon the particular
co-ordinate system used

Fig. 7.2. Typical methods of plotting unlabeled antigen (or ligand) dose inhibition curves, where
P is the concentration of unlabeled antigen (or ligand) and f and b are free and bound labeled
marker. (Taken from R. P. Ekins. 1974. Brit. Med. Bull. 30:3-11.)

binding data, with the possible exception of the logit transformation described below, which lends itself to automatic data computation, no
convincing evidence that they are truly superior exists.

By Logit Transformation

Since the graph of bound antigen versus the log of the total unlabeled antigen concentration is sigmoidal in character (Fig. 7.3), a
sigmoidal transformation results in further linearization of the curve.

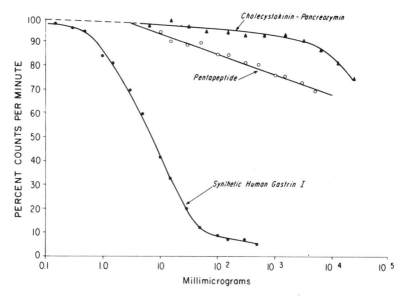

Fig. 7.3. Radioimmunoassay for human gastrin using an antiserum produced against unconjugated human gastrin. Note the nonparallel cross-reacting curve for the pentapeptide containing the same amino acid sequence as the C-terminal portion of gastrin. Cholecystokinin-pancreozymin (CPZ), a larger molecule containing the same pentapeptide sequence in its C-terminal region (Fig. 7.6) produces a less-marked nonparallel cross-reaction. The poorer inhibition of binding by CPZ than the pentapeptide may be due to steric hindrance or differences in tertiary structure when the remainder of the peptide is present. (Taken from W. D. Odell, A. C. Charters, W. D. Davidson, and J. C. Thompson. 1968. J. Clin. Endocr. 28:1840-1842.)

Logit, probit, or arcsine transformations may be used (Rodbard et al., 1968; Rodbard, 1971), and of them the logit is the simplest in terms of the actual mechanics of the calculation. If the percentage of radioactive antigen is designed as Y, then

$$\text{Logit } Y = \log_e \frac{Y}{100 - y}$$

Having calculated logit Y, the ratio of logit Y to bound antigen in un-inhibited controls is then plotted against the log of the unlabeled antigen concentration. The advantage of the logit transformation is that it lends itself readily to computerized programs for calculating the data. Logit log paper suitable for manual computation is also available. The disadvantage of this mathematical treatment is that is accentuates the problem of nonlinearity of residual variance around the regression line. Moreover, since the standard curve is often not a perfect sigmoid curve, displacement of the regression line and possible large errors at the extreme ends of the curve (Challand et al., 1974) may result.

Detailed Analysis
of Binding Inhibition Curves

Once standard, unlabeled antigen inhibition curves for various antisera have been determined, they can be plotted as described under method 1 (counts precipitated versus log unlabeled antigen concentration). This procedure permits a comparison of antisera in regard to the linearity, slope, sensitivity, and other features of their antigen inhibition curves:

1. *Linearity.* As a rule, the inhibition curve is sigmoidal with a central linear segment and curved asymptotic segments at low and high inhibitor concentrations (see Fig. 7.3). In general, useful inhibition data are obtained only in the central linear segment of the curve. Some antisera give inhibition curves that are not linear even in this region, thereby complicating the analysis of the data considerably.

2. *Slope.* Normally the steeper the slope, the better the assay (Yalow and Berson, 1971). The slope in the low-antigen-dose region of the curve is of particular importance if high sensitivity is to be obtained.

3. *Midrange.* A useful parameter in the comparison of antisera is the dose of antigen needed to reduce Ag* binding to 50% of its original level ($B/B_0 = 0.5$, where B and B_0 are the quantities of Ag* bound in the presence and absence of inhibitor). In immunoassays involving large amounts of antibody, the curve may be reasonably steep at high antigen doses but insensitive in the low-antigen-dose regions. For some immunoassay applications, a curve of this type is perfectly satisfactory.

4. *Least detectible dose.* The lowest detectible dose of unlabeled Ag is the smallest dose that causes a statistically significant change in Ag* binding. This factor is determined in part by the standard deviation of binding when unlabeled Ag is absent and by other characteristics of the system. Immunoassay values in samples extracted from tissue often exhibit increased variability or nonspecific inhibitory effects on Ag* binding. As a result, values for least detectible concentrations of Ag need not be the same in buffer as they are in tissue extracts. Since otherwise comparable antisera can vary in their susceptibility to nonspecific inhibition or spontaneous variation in binding, it is desirable to compare their standard inhibition curves in tissue extracts as well as in buffer. Ordinarily no attempt should be made to calculate values in that portion of the low dose range after the curve has broken.

5. *Maximal inhibition.* In general, when large enough quantities of unlabeled antigen are added, radioactive antigen binding is reduced to the nonspecific antigen-binding blank (the binding detected in the assay

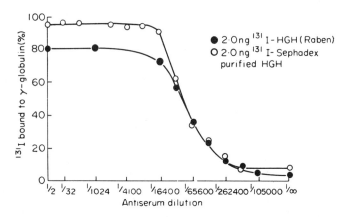

Fig. 7.4. Effect of marker antigen (human-growth hormone, HGH) purity on maximal binding by anti-HGH antibody. ^{131}I-HGH was prepared by iodination of crude (•), and purified (o) preparations of HGH. (Taken from W. M. Hunter. 1973. *In* D. M. Weir (Ed.). Handbook of experimental immunology. Blackwell Scientific Publications, Oxford. pp. 17.1–17.36.)

when antibody is absent). Failure to observe complete inhibition suggests the existence of a contaminating antigen-antibody system (Fig. 7.4).

On rare occasion, marker-binding efficiency actually appears to increase with increases in unlabeled hapten concentration over a portion of the hapten inhibition curve. Obviously such antisera are not useful for immunoassay purposes. This phenomenon has been demonstrated in the DNP-tetrapeptide haptenic system described in Chapter 3, where equilibrium dialysis, fluorescence quenching, and hapten inhibition of precipitation curves all indicated better binding as the molar ratio of hapten-to-antibody sites was increased from 0.1 to 0.4 (Parker et al., 1966). Although the mechanism is unclear, one possibility is a cooperative binding effect in which increasing amounts of hapten produce a conformational change in the antibody, thus increasing its binding affinity. At high ratios of hapten to antibody, most of the antibody would be in the high-affinity configuration and the operational binding affinity would be high. At low hapten-antibody ratios, most of the antibodies would be in their unaltered state and a lower affinity would prevail. Conformational changes in antibody associated with hapten binding have been difficult to demonstrate, but the DNP-tetrapeptide hapten might be better able than most haptens to direct a selective reorientation of the antibody molecule because of its size. Aggregation of hapten molecules as the hapten concentration is increased with improved binding of the aggregates is another possibility that must be considered. Regardless of the explanation, the effect is of considerable interest because of its possible relationship to so-called reverse-slope inhibition curves occasionally seen with antibodies to ACTH (Matsukura et al., 1971), calcitonin (Niederer, 1974), and 3-carboxymethylmorphine (S. Spector, personal communication), where, in selected segments of the ligand inhibition curve, increasing amounts of unlabeled inhibitor actually result in better rather than poorer binding of marker. With ACTH and calcitonin, the effect is obtained with labeled marker alone, indicating that it is not due to differences in immunoreactivity of the labeled and unlabeled antigen. In the calcitonin system it is not seen with univalent antibody fragments, thus suggesting that an ability to form sizable aggregates is involved and hence a different mechanism than that suggested for the DNP-tetrapeptide hapten. It is possible that when multivalent antibody molecules react with antigen, they alter its three-dimensional structure, creating new areas for binding on the antigen. Regardless of the explanation, most antisera to ACTH and calcitonin do not exhibit anomalous binding, and so it is possible to measure these substances by immunoassay.

ANALYSIS OF CROSS-REACTIVITY

One of the most important criteria for a useful antiserum is that it be as free as possible of immunological cross-reactivity for related antigens also present in tissue extracts. Cross-reactivity is evaluated by running simultaneous, separate standard curves with the homologous and cross-reacting antigens. It is also useful to see what happens to the standard curve for homologous antigen when various quantities of cross-reacting antigen are also present—particularly when the approximate level of cross-reacting antigen present in tissue is known. Several types of cross-reactivity patterns may be seen.

Complete Cross-reactivity

The inhibition curve with the cross-reacting antigen may parallel that with the homologous antigen over the full inhibition range (e.g., from 5% inhibition to > 90% inhibition). This situation indicates complete cross-reactivity. As a rule, a cross-reacting antigen that gives a parallel inhibition curve with one antiserum will usually give parallel curves with other antisera, but this is not always the case. Even if it were, the relative inhibition observed with the different antisera can vary by as much as two orders of magnitude.

Incomplete Cross-reactivity

A cross-reacting antigen may inhibit effective inhibition in the low dose range but fail to inhibit maximally at high concentrations (Fig. 7.5).

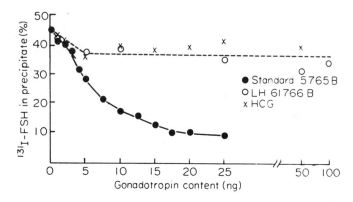

Fig. 7.5. Inhibition of FSH marker binding to anti-FSH antibody by FSH (5765B), LH, and HCG. Note the inhibition at low concentrations of LH and HCG with failure to see increasing inhibition at higher concentrations of these proteins. (Taken from J. R. Ryan, and C. Faiman. 1968. *In* M. Margoulies (Ed.). Protein and polypeptide hormones. Excerpta Medica, International Congress Series 161, Amsterdam. p. 131.)

Consequently, only a portion of the antibodies present is cross-reactive. Another form of incomplete cross-reactivity is evidenced by inhibition curves that fail to parallel the curve with homologous antigen (Fig. 7.3), as shown by gastrin and pancreozymin-cholecytokinin, which have a common C-terminal pentapeptide (Fig. 7.6).

As a rule, when a series of cross-reacting antigens are compared,

a 1 2 3 4 5 6 7 8 9 10 11 12 13 14 15 16
   Lys-Ala-Pro-Ser-Gly-Arg-Val-Ser-Met-Ile-Lys-Asn-Leu-Gln-Ser-Leu–

   17 18 19 20 21 22 23 24 25 26   27   28   29 30 31 32 33
   Asp-Pro-Ser-His-Arg-Ile-Ser-Asp-Arg-Asp-Tyr(SO₃)-Met-│Gly-Trp-Met-Asp-Phe(NH₂)│

b Glu-Gly-Pro-Tyr-Met-Glu-Glu-Glu-Glu-Glu-Ala-Tyr(SO₃)-│Gly-Trp-Met-Asp-Phe(NH₂)│

   1 2 3 4 5 6 7 8 9 10 11   12   13 14 15 16 17

Regions of homology are shown in the box

Fig. 7.6. Amino acid sequence of porcine (a) pancreozymincholecystokinin and (b) gastrin II. (Taken from S. R. Bloom. 1974. Brit. Med. Bull. 30:62-67.)

they retain their rank order of effectiveness as inhibitors with different antisera. However, exceptions occur, as noted in immunoassays for steroids (Hunter, 1973). These variations can be logically explained by the existence of antibodies that differ in the area of the steroid ring to which they are adapted. Such a reordering of cross-reactivity is less likely although theoretically possible with protein antigens.

STATISTICAL AND QUALITY CONTROL CONSIDERATIONS

Rodbard and his colleagues have discussed statistical aspects of radioimmunoassays in detail (Rodbard et al., 1968; Rodbard, 1971). In general, the variation between replicate tubes in the same assay is on the order of 2 to 5%. Cotes et al. (1969) conducted an interesting study of interassay variation in insulin measurements within the same laboratory and found a range between 88 to 114% in the best laboratory and 50 to 202% in the worst laboratory. Useful quality control checks for determining the basis for interassay variation include the specific activity of the marker, the quantity of marker added to assay tubes, the level of nonspecific marker binding, the maximal level of marker binding, marker tissue incubation controls, and the slope and relative sensitivity of the standard curve. In several recent cooperative studies, laboratories using locally raised antibodies have exchanged unknown samples and compared their immunoassay results (Cotes et al., 1969; Bogdanove et al., 1971). In general, the agreement was surprisingly good.

AUTOMATION

In the past few years there has been considerable progress in speeding up the assay process. With simple, inexpensive, rapid-dispensing equipment in a double antibody system, a single technician can process from 500 to 1,000 samples/day. Undoubtedly future trends will be toward increasing automation and large, centralized, immunossay-processing laboratories.

REPRESENTATIVE ASSAY SENSITIVITIES

Representative assay sensitivities are given in Table 7.1. Note that sensitivities in the low femtomole range are achieved in most protein and polypeptide hormone assays and that high sensitivities are also obtained in hapten immunoassays.

Table 7.1

Representative sensitivities for protein, polypeptide, and hapten immunoassays.

	Reported sensitivity	
Immune system	Picograms	Phentomoles
Parathormone	4	0.4
Placental lactogen	50	2
Growth hormone	80	4
Gastrin	10	5
ACTH	5	1
Glucagon	20	6
Angiotensin	10	10
Thyroxine	100	130
Digoxin	25	30
Morphine	200	700
Cyclic AMP	80	250
Cyclic GMP	10	30

Based on typical sensitivities rather than the maximal sensitivities reported in the literature. Modified from Appendix I of Jaffe and Behrman (1974).

SUMMARY

1. As a rule, the radioimmunoassay itself is used as the primary means of evaluating antisera. Once antisera with intermediate or high titers have been identified, they are systemically compared in regard to maximal sensitivity, steepness, linearity, and reproducibility of standard inhibition curves in tissue samples and buffer. Sera that best meet the overall requirements of the immunoassay are selected.

2. Variables in the immunoassay include total incubation volume, buffer, quantity of antibody and radioactive antigen, time and order of addition of reactants, temperature and total duration of incubation, mode of separation of free and bound antigen, and whether bound or free antigen is counted.

3. When a highly sensitive immunoassay is needed, careful studies on the effect of buffer pH and ionic strength on assay sensitivity and specificity can be helpful in optimizing the assay.

4. A minimum of 5,000 to 10,000 cpm of radioactive antigen per individual assay tube is used in order to obtain adequate levels of bound-antigen radioactivity.

5. Dilutions of antibody that bind 30 to 50% of the radioactive antigen are commonly optimal. In general, the antibody need not be purified before assay. Requirements for antibody in tissue may be somewhat higher than they are in buffer.

6. Dilutions of tissue extracts that bring the level of immunoinhibitory activity into the range of the standard curve are used. It is sometimes desirable to divide tissue extracts into several portions and assay large and small aliquots. Depending on the assay, partial purification or concentration of antigen in tissue extracts may be necessary before immunologic analysis.

7. The antigen content of tissue samples is calculated from the standard antigen inhibition curve. A number of graphical methods for expressing and calculating radioimmunoassay data exist. For manually calculated data, a plot of precipitated counts versus log antigen dose is probably as satisfactory as any other. For automated calculation of data, a logit transformation, which further linearizes the standard inhibition curve, can be used.

8. Useful quality control measurements for determining the basis for interassay variation include the specific activity of the marker, the quantity of marker added to assay tubes, the level of nonspecific marker binding, the maximal level of marker binding, marker-tissue incubation curves, and the slope and relative sensitivity of the standard inhibition curve.

Chapter 8

Separation of Antibody-Bound and Free Antigen

The final step in a radioimmunoassay involves the measurement of bound or free antigen. In most immunoassay systems such measurement requires that bound and free antigen be separated physically. Ideally, the separation procedure should be applicable to the simultaneous processing of a large number of immunoassay samples. In addition, separation should be achieved without undue dissociation of preformed antigen-antibody complexes or reequilibration to form new complexes. Numerous methods are available; they exploit differences between free and bound antigen in immunological reactivity, molecular size, electrophoretic mobility, salt or organic solvent solubility, or absorbability to solid-phase reagents.

The choice of a method for separating free and bound antigen depends on a number of factors, including the solubility and absorption properties of the radioactive antigen, the requirements of the assay in terms of speed and reproducibility, and the susceptibility of the antigen-antibody system to dissociation during the separation. Once enough initial screening has been done to narrow the choice to one of several separation procedures, they can be directly compared under the operational conditions of the assay (e.g., in measurements of tissue samples), and the one that meets the requirements of the assay best can be selected.

THE DOUBLE-ANTIBODY METHOD

In general, the concentrations of antigen-antibody complexes present in sensitive immunoassays are low, and precipitation does not occur unless a coprecipitating system is present.

The double-antibody method, which is perhaps the most widely used of the separation methods, was first utilized as a coprecipitating system

156

for immunoassay measurements by Utiger, Parker, and Daughaday (1962). The method depends on the ability of anti-immunoglobulin antibodies to bind to soluble antigen-antibody complexes and cause precipitation of the entire complex, separating any bound radiolabeled antigen that is present. The anti-immunoglobulin antibody is obtained by immunizing a second species with purified "nonspecific" gamma globulin from the species serving as the source of first antibody. Second antibodies produced in this way are largely directed toward antigenic regions on the immunizing gamma globulin outside the antibody-combining sites, explaining their ability to combine with molecules of first antibody already attached to antigen. Thus goat, guinea pig, or horse antirabbit gamma globulin can all be used to precipitate rabbit gamma globulin; and if the rabbit gamma globulin is from an immunized animal, the system can be used to determine antigen binding. The precipitation is carried out in second antibody excess as determined by varying the concentration of second antibody until maximal precipitation of radioactive antigen is obtained.

As a rule, the first antibody reaction is initiated before the second antibody is introduced. First antibody, unlabeled antigen, and radiolabeled antigen are preincubated for a few minutes to up to 72 hours, the second antibody is added, and the incubation is continued for another 4 to 48 hours at 4°C. After adequate time for precipitation, precipitated complexes are isolated by centrifugation and washed. Bound radiolabel is determined by counting the washed precipitation directly or is determined from the quantity of radioactivity in the original supernatant (by difference). The time required for optimal precipitation in the second antibody step depends on the relative concentrations of first antibody gamma globulin and second antibody. In some systems preformed first antibody-second antibody complexes bind effectively to antigen, permitting a more rapid assay, albeit with some diminution in sensitivity. However, this procedure is not always possible; when hepatitis B antigen is assayed, formation of the double-antibody complex impairs antigen bonding, and the addition of second antibody must be delayed for at least several hours (Aach et al., 1971).

To date, double-antibody precipitation appears to have been the most widely applicable method for separating free and bound antigen. Very sensitive measurements are possible with a high degree of reproducibility in a large number of antigen-antibody systems. There has been concern about the time required for development of macroscopic precipitates and the possibility of reequilibration in the first antigen-antibody reaction, but, in practice, it has not been a problem. Once the second antibody has been added, there is a slowing of the first antibody reaction but little or no evidence that preformed antigen-antibody complexes actually dissociate. Indeed, it is possible that appropriately chosen second antibodies increase complex stability. Although it has been argued that the necessity of adding second antibody is a major inconvenience, this step can be done rapidly with semiautomatic dispensing equipment. The time requirement for obtaining adequate precipitation in double-antibody immunoassays is a drawback only if very rapid measurements are needed, and this factor is usually an unimportant one.

If the first antibody has a very low titer (dilutions of 1:50 or less), the expenditure of second antibody is prohibitive and other methods must be used. On a per molecule basis, it takes about 8 to 10 molecules of second antibody to precipitate a single molecule of first antibody; but the requirement is actually much more severe, since all the nonspecific gamma globulin present must also be precipitated before true second antibody excess is achieved.*

Despite the broad applicability of the double-antibody method, a number of inherent pitfalls should be noted:

1. In measurements in human sera, the second antibody should be carefully screened for cross-reactions with human gamma globulin.

2. The diluted antiserum containing the first antibody must have a high enough total γ-globulin concentration (usually 2 to 5 μg/ml) to give a macroscopic precipitate when excess second antibody is added (Parker, 1972b). Since the concentration of γ-globulin in serum is normally about 10 mg/ml, difficulties in obtaining adequate precipitation do not arise, as a rule, until dilutions of antiserum that exceed 1:1,000 are reached (0.1 ml of a 1:1,000 dilution of an antiserum in a final volume of 0.3 ml would contain roughly 3 μg of γ-globulin/ml). With more highly diluted antisera, carrier serum or γ-globulin can be added to keep precipitation at the desired level.

3. Because of the minimal quantities of protein precipitated, it is necessary to maintain samples at 4°C during washing so as to avoid solubilizing precipitates. This step is particularly important when large numbers of tubes are being processed. Larger quantities of precipitate are avoided in order to minimize expenditure of second antibody and nonspecific adherence of radioantigen to precipitates.

4. Occasionally a preparation of second antibody with an apparently adequate precipitin titer gives unreliable results in the immunoassay. Certain antisera give ineffective precipitation of radioactivity when too large an excess of antibody is present, either because of a floculation-

---

* It has been suggested that the requirement for second antibody can be reduced by utilizing low concentrations of ammonium sulfate (Ratcliffe, 1974).

type precipitin curve or the formation of a less-adherent precipitate. This condition is more prominent with horse, sheep, or goat antisera than with rabbit antisera.

5. Interference to precipitation is sometimes seen when tissue extracts are measured, and it may be desirable to double or triple the amount of second antibody as a hedge against such an effect. Whatever dilution is selected, the ability of second antibody to produce maximal precipitation of radioantigen in tissue samples must be directly verified. Lipid and fibrin also interfere with precipitate formation and should be removed by centrifugation prior to the assay.

SALT AND SOLVENT PRECIPITATION

Salt or organic solvent precipitation is another useful technique for the separation of antigen-antibody complexes from free antigen. The method depends on the relative ease with which γ-globulin and antigen-antibody complexes are precipitated from aqueous solution by sulfate salts and water-miscible organic solvents. Ammonium sulfate precipitation is the most widely used salting-out method. It has been employed in the development of immunoassays to digitoxin, cyclic AMP, morphine, the prostaglandins, lysine vasopressin, oxytocin, and arginine vasopressin (Parker, 1972b), all of which are soluble in 2 M ammonium sulfate (approximately 50% of saturation), and is also applicable to measurement of protein-antigen binding (Farr, 1958). Unbound immunoglobulins and antigen-antibody complexes are precipitated almost quantitatively at 4°C in 1.6 M ammonium sulfate (about 40% of saturation), provided that the preprecipitation protein concentration is in a suitable range. The precipitation is carried out in the presence of carrier serum or gamma globulin (preferably from the same animal species as the antibody) at a final gamma globulin concentration of approximately 200 to 500 $\mu g/ml$. After preliminary incubation of unlabeled antigen, labeled antigen, and antibody, 0.6 to 1.0 volumes of an ice-cold saturated solution of ammonium sulfate in water are added, with rapid mixing to avoid zone effects. Failure to mix immediately is an important source of variation in assay results. After 20 to 30 minutes at 4°C, the precipitates are isolated by centrifugation, washed with 40% ammonium sulfate, and counted. In scintillation mixtures used for counting ^3H and ^{14}C, the residual salt usually precipitates, but ordinarily it does not affect counting efficiency adversely. Advantages of the method include speed, reproducibility, and relative lack of expense. However, the method is not as widely applicable as the double-antibody technique, for it is often impossible to find conditions that permit the complete separation of bound and free antigen. Many antigens are insoluble at ammonium sulfate concentrations of 40% or below, and in this case other methods must be used. Another potential problem is the high binding blanks that sometimes arise with radiolabeled antigens that tend to adhere nonspecifically to precipitates.

Nonspecific Absorbents

Free antigen can be absorbed from solution by a variety of solid particles. When antibody is present, absorption of antigen is reduced, providing the basis for a competitive binding assay. Charcoal is the most widely used absorbent. After the antigen-antibody system has been allowed to equilibrate for the desired period of time, charcoal is added. After a variable, usually brief period of time the mixture is centrifuged, and either the charcoal or the supernatant is counted. Wood charcoals with particle sizes of less than 60 μ are generally used. In the original method the charcoal was coated with a dextran of defined molecular size (Herbert, 1969) in order to partially occlude the pores of the charcoal so that proteins and polypeptide antigens that were larger than the openings (or pores) would be excluded from the charcoal and smaller antigens would be absorbed. Later evidence indicates that dextran is not needed, provided that sufficient amounts of whole serum are present ($>$ 10%; vol:vol). The charcoal method is not only simple and inexpensive, but rapid measurements are possible as well. For example, levels of digitalis in blood can be obtained within 30 to 60 minutes (assuming that the blood is processed immediately after it was drawn; see Fig. 8.1) (Smith et al., 1969; Oliver et al., 1971). However, the method does not seem to apply to every antigen-antibody system; bound as well as free antigen may absorb to the charcoal or the affinity of the charcoal for free antigen may be so high that the antigen-antibody reaction is affected. Another factor is that unless supernatant solutions are rapidly and carefully separated from the charcoal, erratic results may be obtained. For this reason, it is important that the assay be limited to an easily manageable number of tubes.

Other nonspecific solid-phase absorbents, in addition to charcoal, include cellulose, silicates (Quso G-32, talc, Fluorasil), glass or plastic test tubes, and ion exchange resins.

Immunologically Specific Absorbents

As noted, either the antigen or the antibody can be insolubilized through a covalent or noncovalent bond onto a solid particle, tube, disk, fiber, or belt and used later as an immunologically specific reagent in the

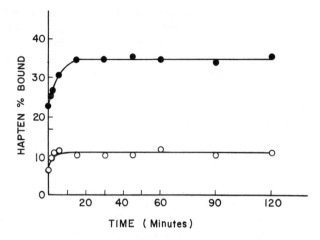

Fig. 8.1. Rate of equilibration between antidigoxin antibody and ^3H digoxin in plasma at 4° C. ^3H digoxin was added at time zero. Closed circles, plasma not containing digoxin; open circles, plasma containing digoxin, 1 ngm/ml. The expected reduction in the percent hapten bound to antibody is seen. However, there is no apparent difference in the time required to reach equilibrium. (Taken from G. C. Oliver, B. M. Parker, and C. W. Parker. 1971. Amer. J. Med. 51:186-192.)

immunoassay. This procedure removes one of the immunologically specific reactants in the assay from solution, thus facilitating the separation of free and bound antigen (or antibody). Covalently bound reactants are preferred because of the reduced likelihood of solubilization of antigen or antibody from the particle. Covalent bond formation is generally accomplished by a two-step procedure in which the particle is reacted with bifunctional activating agent and then exposed to the antigen or antibody under conditions favoring conjugation. In conjugations involving antibody, ideally, gamma globulin fractions rather than whole serum should be used in order to minimize binding of extraneous proteins to the partide. Activation is most commonly accomplished with cyanogen bromide or bromoacetyl bromide. Alternatively, stable azide or aromatic amine residues can be introduced onto particules and activated just prior to the introduction of the protein, or particles containing primary aliphatic amino or carboxyl groups can be combined with antibody or antigen with one of the coupling agents described in Chapter 2. Particles that have been shown to be satisfactory for routine immunoassay applications include agarose, Sephadex, polyacrylamide, and cellulose. Unfortunately, it is not possible at present to single out a particular particle or method of conjugation as clearly superior to the others. Indeed, considering the large number of different antigens that might be assayed by solid-phase methods, it would be somewhat surprising if a single system turned out to be universally applicable.

Solid-phase systems involving polystyrene tubes coated with a thin film of antibody by nonspecific absorption have also been used successfully (Catt, 1970). In this procedure dilutions of the antibody are incubated in tubes at a weakly alkaline pH, after which the tubes are washed. Under these conditions the antibody is bound sufficiently firmly to the tube to permit the tube to be used as a solid-phase absorbent.

Such systems have the advantage of simplicity and rapidity. However, it is sometimes difficult to achieve reproducible levels of binding. The establishment of equilibrium, while rapid in some systems, requires continuous mixing over a period of many hours in others. If the problem is not recognized and dealt with effectively, the assay may produce erratic results, which is perhaps the major complaint about solid-phase systems. The achievement of adequate sensitivity may also present problems, depending to a large extent on the antigen-antibody system and the method of conjugation. Some solid-phase assays are significantly less sensitive than the corresponding soluble assay system. For example, in immunological measurements of gastrin, conjugation of antibody to bromoacetyl cellulose resulted in a fourfold fall in its average affinity for antigen (Rehfeld and Stadil, 1973). In some assay systems even this modest fall in binding affinity might be unacceptable.

Electrophoresis, Chromatoelectrophoresis, and Thin-Layer Chromatography

Electrophoresis or chromatoelectrophoresis has been used extensively by Berson, Yalow, and their colleagues (Yalow and Berson, 1960; Yalow and Berson, 1970a). In this method soluble, previously equilibrated mixtures containing antibody and labeled and unlabeled antigen are applied to chromatography paper and subjected to an electrophoretic field. Free and antibody-bound antigen are separated on the basis of electrophoretic mobility and the tendency of certain proteins to adhere to cellulose when they are not bound by antibody (e.g., insulin, parathormone, ACTH, and growth hormone). The distribution of radiolabeled antigen is evaluated in an automatic strip counter. For antigen-antibody systems in which poor separation is obtained on paper, starch gel is sometimes a useful substitute. The major advantage of this method is that it routinely detects incubation damage to the radioactive antigen, and separate antigen damage control tubes are not needed. On the other hand, it is laborious, expensive, not subject to automation, requires considerable cold-room space, and the electric current needed is a potential hazard to other investigators working in the same area. Moreover, there is variation in individual batches of chromatography paper, requiring reevaluation of the electrochromatography conditions from time to time. Electrophoretic separation techniques employing other solid supports suffer from many of the same disadvantages. Thin-layer chromatography systems that do not utilize an electric current are not hazardous, but they have limited sample-volume capacities and may be mechanically complex.

MOLECULAR SIEVE FILTRATION OR EQUILIBRATION

Filtration through a molecular sieve can be used to separate free and antibody-bound antigen. Suitable sieves include Sephadex, agarose, and specially prepared glass beads, the choice depending on the molecular weight and absorption properties of the antigen. Major drawbacks include the need to utilize an individual column for each immunoassay sample and the extra time required for careful monitoring of columns if free and bound antigen migrate close together. As a result, the method has a low-sample capacity, and other methods are far more preferable when large numbers of samples are being processed.

Gel equilibration is a potentially more useful method, although thus far it has only been applied on a limited basis. A gel that is permeable to free antigen is allowed to equilibrate with a solution of radioactive antigen at the beginning of the assay. Antibody with or without unlabeled antigen is added, and because antigen-antibody complexes are unable to enter the gel, a new equilibrium is established (Ratcliffe, 1974). The gels are separated by gravity or centrifugation, and the supernatant is counted. The method has been utilized commercially in the Thyopac 4 Kit.

SUMMARY

1. The final step in a radioimmunoassay is the determination of free or bound antigen. As a rule, this step requires that free and bound antigen be separated physically. (Several immunoassay systems in which separation is not necessary are discussed in Chapter 5.)

2. Free and bound antigen may be separated in the immunoassay by differences in immunological reactivity, salt or organic solvent solubility, electrophoretic mobility, molecular size, or absorbability to solid-phase reagents.

3. The choice of a method for separating free and bound antigen depends on a number of factors, including the solubility and absorption properties of the radioactive antigen, the requirements of the assay in terms of speed and reproducibility, and the susceptibility of preformed antigen-antibody complexes to dissociation during the separation. Once the choice has been narrowed to several apparently suitable separation

procedures, they can be compared operationally in the assay, and the one that best meets the requirements of the assay can be selected.

4. The double-antibody method has the advantage of broad applicability, sensitivity, and reproducibility. Salt or solvent precipitation or nonspecific absorption methods permit more rapid (and at times equally sensitive) measurements and, in general, utilize relatively inexpensive reagents. Specific immunoabsorbent systems may also lend themselves to rapid and sensitive measurements. Chromatoelectrophoresis or gel filtration separation methods are more laborious and less desirable in general.

Chapter 9

Problems in Immunoassay Measurements in Tissue Samples

INTRODUCTION

It comes as something of a rude awakening to neophyte or even experienced investigators to find that radioimmunoassay systems that give sensitive and reproducible standard curves in buffer sometimes produce erratic or even erroneous results in tissue. This situation may be manifested (a) as a failure to find the expected increase in antigen content when known quantities of unlabeled antigen are added to the assay, (b) by an inability to demonstrate the expected changes in tissue antigen content in response to reliable pharmacologic stimuli, or (c) by a failure to show proportionality between the quantity of tissue extracted and the measured quantity of antigen. Depending on the tissue, it may be vital to extract and partially purify the antigen prior to immunoassay, but the extraction process itself may lead to decreases or increases in antigen content or to the introduction of substances that nonspecifically interfere with immunologic reactivity. In many immunoassay systems careful attention to the problem of optimal tissue extraction is as important as having immunologically specific reagents. Unfortunately, each new antigen-antibody system, and, to a lesser extent, each new tissue, is somewhat of an individual problem, depending on the quantity of antigen to be measured, the probability of enzymatic destruction of antigen, and the molecular properties of the antigen in terms of stability and ease of separation from interfering substances. In addition, the binding properties of the antibody are important. Fortunately, enough knowledge is available from carefully studied immunoassay systems to enable the investigator to anticipate the general kinds of problems that may arise. Many are not unique to immunoassay measurements but are sources of difficulty regardless of the analytical procedure being used. This chapter will consider what the possible sources of error are and how they may be detected and circumvented.

DESTRUCTION OR FORMATION OF ANTIGEN

When measurements are made in plasma, it is necessary to separate the plasma from formed elements of the blood. This procedure requires that blood that has been prevented from clotting be centrifuged or filtered. Alternatively, serum or whole-blood extracts may be utilized. The latter are obtained by freezing the blood or extracting directly by the addition of an organic solvent or a protein-denaturing agent, such as trichloroacetic acid, without prior separation of cells. All three procedures have drawbacks. Extraction of whole blood will almost certainly disrupt the cells, which will then discharge whatever antigen they contain into the extracellular milieu. The separation of plasma inevitably delays the establishment of protein denaturation or protein separation procedures that may be needed to inactivate or remove plasma enzymes. For many drugs and circulating proteins, this situation poses no special problem, and valid analytical results are obtained even when special precautions are not taken to maintain blood samples at 4°C and carry out the separation of plasma promptly. Measurements of plasma polypeptide hormones, such as bradykinin, PTH, ACTH, angiotensin I, angiotensin II, and insulin, are another matter. These substances are highly susceptible to degradation by proteolytic enzymes in blood. Indeed, Goodfriend and Odya (1974) have estimated that the half life of circulating bradykinin is on the order of 1 minute. Rapid degradation is also a potential problem with cyclic nucleotides, which are converted by phosphodiesterases in plasma to the corresponding 5′ nucleotides, with histamine, which can be broken down by plasma histaminases, and with catecholamines and prostaglandins, which are subject to both enzymatic and chemical breakdown. Obviously the stability of the antigen is an important factor in immunoassays involving blood, and unusual care may be needed to avoid degradation of antigen during initial processing.

Procedures used for obtaining samples free of formed elements of the blood with little or no degradation by plasma enzymes vary with the substance and the investigator. Rapid inactivation processes that have been recommended in making bradykinin measurements in blood include an initial ethanol, hexadimethrine-EDTA, or acid (perchloric, formic, or hydrochloric) extraction. Bradykinin is strongly basic, and absorption to a cation exchange resin, followed by washing to remove serum enzymes and elution of absorbed bradykinin, has been employed in an attempt to stabilize the oligopeptide during the initial extraction phase (Talamo et al., 1969). However, the process has serious disadvantages. As discussed below, it is just as important to avoid new antigen formation during extraction as it is to prevent the degradation of preformed antigen, and this feature is particularly important in the kinin system. The resin method is one of the extraction procedures that fails to accomplish this goal, presumably because contact of the blood with the resin surface activates kinin-forming enzymes (Goodfriend and Odya, 1974). The multiplicity of extraction procedures for bradykinin is an indication of the lack of general agreement as to what procedure is optimal. Regardless of the extraction method used, it is important to use siliconized, precooled catheters and syringes to help avoid stimulation of the kinin system while the blood is being collected.

Even assuming that the plasma sample is treated to inactivate degradative enzymes, low levels of enzyme activity may persist or be reintroduced when the antibody is added (for most enzymes, this situation can be avoided by using purified gamma globulin fractions rather than crude antisera). In addition, partially purified serum albumins are widely used in immunoassay diluent solutions as a means of reducing nonspecific binding and should be considered as a source of proteolytic enzymes. Since low levels of proteolytic activity are difficult to exclude, it is often desirable to introduce a proteolytic enzyme inhibitor into the sample, usually at the time of the initial extraction. Goodfriend and Odya (1974) list 15 enzyme inhibitors that have been used with varying degrees of effectiveness to forestall antigen inactivation or formation in the kinin-bradykinin system. They include heavy metals, small-molecular-weight competitive enzyme inhibitors, high-molecular-weight enzyme inhibitors (e.g., soybean trypsin inhibitor), and chelating agents. These enzyme inhibitors can have important effects in the immunoassay. The choice of an inactivation procedure may be influenced to some extent by the antiserum, since antisera vary in the extent to which antigen binding is affected by the various enzyme inhibitors. Such variation can be seen even within a single antigen-antibody system. Despite the addition of inhibitor, residual enzyme activity may persist, thus creating a potential source of error in assay results. And since the residual enzyme activity can vary from sample to sample, it may be difficult to compare results in different individuals. Under these conditions it is necessary to include a screening procedure for marker degradation as one of the routine controls in the immunoassay. It is done by incubating marker and sample together under the usual immunoassay conditions and looking for physicochemical or immunological evidence of marker degradation. The marker is chromatographed or precipitated with excess antibody to obtain a value for maximal marker binding and compared with the control (nonpreincubated) marker. If evidence of residual proteolytic activity is found, its effects in the immunoassay may be minimized by the use of more dilute plasma samples or by keeping the temperature and total time of the assay to a minimum. Alternatively, a different or more elaborate preliminary extraction procedure or new enzyme inhibitors may be tried.

It should be emphasized that any extraction procedure that is used may introduce new artifacts in the immunoassay. For example, trichloroacetic acid or trichloroacetic acid salts may interfere with antibody binding. Although extraction with ether can be used to remove most of the trichloroacetic acid, possible effects of peroxides in the ether or residual ether itself must be considered. Effects of salts or unneutralized acid in the original blood or extracting medium are magnified if the sample is concentrated prior to its incorporation in the immunoassay, and frequently some form of desalting is needed. Other potential problems in extraction include denaturation or degradation of antigen, losses of antigen due to nonspecific adherence to glassware or precipitated proteins, or actual creation of antigen during extraction. As noted, for oligopeptides like bradykinin, angiotensin I, and angiotensin II, which are derived from precursor proteins or polypeptides present in blood, the possibility must be considered that part of what is being measured is created during the collection or extraction of the blood or even at the time of the radioimmunoassay. Cells present in blood may also serve as a biosynthetic source of antigen, especially if the blood is allowed to clot at 37°C to obtain serum. In this case, prostaglandins, serotonin, histamine, and other substances may be released from leukocytes or platelets and contribute to the total serum value. With prostaglandins, which are enzymatically generated in platelets and leukocytes from lipid precursors, this difficulty can be avoided by maintaining the blood at 4°C during processing (Jaffe et. al., 1973). With histamine and serotonin, which are synthesized and stored in their biologically active form inside cells, it is necessary to avoid traumatizing or otherwise activating the cells, and the simple precaution of avoiding incubating the cells at 37°C and obtaining plasma rather than serum will not be completely effective. However, the combined use of low temperature, gentle separation procedures, and the incorporation of a chelating agent for calcium in the medium will usually reduce release to only a few percent of the total cellular histamine content of the cells, particularly if the blood is processed promptly. In addition to antigen formed or released by conventional metabolic processes, antigen may be formed nonenzymatically during exposure of the tissue to extremes of heat or pH. For example, $cGMP$ is formed nonenzymatically when tissue samples containing GTP and divalent cations are heated to 100°C (Kimura and Murad, 1974).

The problems that arise in extracting the antigen may be even more severe in tissue than they are in blood. Measured values for pharmacologically active substances that turn over rapidly inside the cell can fluctuate markedly, depending on how the sample is processed. For example, the apparent concentration of cAMP in heart tissue changes, depending on whether the sample is processed by trichloroacetic acid extraction, rapid freezing in liquid nitrogen, or by placing the tissue between cooled metal blocks. Significant destruction of cAMP can probably occur in periods as short as 1 to 3 seconds (Mayer et al., 1974). With substances present at very low concentrations in tissue, it may be difficult to decide what the true value is. Nor can it be assumed that extraction methods that are satisfactory in one tissue are necessarily adequate in another. This point is true for cAMP measurements in tissue where direct boiling and sonication may or may not give values that correspond to those obtained by other methods.

Apart from inactivation during extraction or in the assay itself, optimal methods for storage of extracts should be considered. cAMP and cGMP measurements may be falsely low if the tissue or tissue extract is not maintained at $-70°C$ or below during storage. Labile proteins and small molecular weight drugs that are subject to oxidation or reduction, such as the catecholamines or prostaglandins, may undergo gradual losses in antigenic reactivity even when stored under apparently optimal conditions, particularly if preliminary partial purification is not carried out prior to storage.

FACTORS IN TISSUE OR SERUM INTERFERING WITH THE BINDING OF ANTIGEN TO ANTIBODY

As noted earlier, extraction procedures that alter the ionic strength, pH, or divalent cation content of the sample or that carry over interfering substances from the original tissue may have adverse effects on antibody binding and interfere in the immunoassay. The result may be reduced assay sensitivity or alterations in the kinetics of the antigen-antibody reaction, leading to different incubation requirements in the assay. In addition, spurious results may be obtained. When the sample contains interfering substances and the standard antigen inhibition curve is measured in their absence, the absolute values for antigen in the sample will be meaningless even though some indication may be obtained of the *relative* antigen content of different samples. Where samples contain variable amounts of interfering substances, even the apparent relative antigen content may be misleading. For example, immunoassay measurements in urine are affected by wide variations in urine osmolality, pH, and urea content (Parker, 1972b). If only a very small quantity of urine is needed to make the measurement, the final immunoassay sample will be so dilute that no interference will occur. Otherwise preliminary extraction prior to assay will generally be necessary. No ironclad rules can be given, since different antigen-antibody systems and even individual antisera within a given system vary considerably in their susceptibility to nonspecific interference.

Another type of interference involves a competition between the antibody and proteins present in blood or tissue that have affinity for the antigen. Many therapeutic agents are bound reversibly to serum albumins, and although the affinity of the interaction is usually less than 1×10^6 liters/mole, because of the large quantities of albumin in blood, significant competition between albumin and antibody may still occur. Competitive binding to albumin is more likely to be a problem with hydrophobic or anionic drugs that tend to undergo relatively high affinity interactions with albumin. In the initial immunoassay for a cardiac glucoside, digitoxin was measured after extraction of plasma or serum with an organic solvent (Oliver et al., 1968). The method was sufficiently rapid to be useful in emergency clinical situations and had the sensitivity needed to measure pharmacologic as well as toxic levels of the drug, but the extraction portion of the procedure did somewhat slow the rate of sample processing. When high-affinity antidigitoxin antibodies ($K_a \sim 10^{10}$ liters/mole) became available (Smith et al., 1969; Oliver et al., 1971), the antibody competed sufficiently well with albumin ($K_a \sim 10^5$ liters/mole) that useful measurements could be made even without a preliminary extraction, thereby increasing the rapidity and convenience of the assay. Nonetheless, immunoassay measurements in the presence of competing serum proteins have important built-in pitfalls, particularly if rapid measurements are being made. Depending on the thermodynamic and kinetic dissociation constants for the drug albumin interaction, a portion of the drug is still bound to the albumin, and this portion is exaggerated when short incubation conditions are used. Under these nonequilibrium conditions the way in which samples are handled must be carefully standardized, and some variation in results, depending on serum albumin levels or concurrent use of drugs that bind competitively to albumin, can be anticipated.

Many agents cannot be measured without a preliminary extraction—for example, various prostaglandins circulate in low concentrations tightly bound to serum albumin. However, in prostaglandin immunoassays, the requirement for extraction is not as onerous as it sounds, since the extracts can be utilized directly in a simple chromatographic procedure that cleanly separates the individual prostaglandin groups and considerably enhances the information obtainable by radioimmunoassay (see Chapter 9) (Jaffe et al., 1973).

Not all the binding interference in radioimmunoassay measurements involves small molecular weight ligands and albumins. The blood contains proteins with binding affinities for a variety of naturally occurring hormones, including thyroxin and many different steroid hormones. As discussed in Chapter 10, these proteins bind the various hormones sufficiently well that they can be used as substitutes for antibody in competitive binding measurements. When a conventional immunoassay system is being used, the binding proteins are a problem because their levels are not fixed in blood, and therefore they interfere to a variable extent in the immunoassay. Depending on the immunoassay system involved, extraction may be necessary to eliminate this difficulty.

Specific binding protein or albumin effects on immunoassays can be anticipated and dealt with on a routine basis. Unexpected difficulties may arise if a binding protein not normally present in the blood appears. Although not a common problem, it does represent still another potential source of error in routine immunoassay measurements. The competing protein may be an antibody formed by the host in response to previous treatment with the protein or drug. Antibody formation can occur in children receiving foreign protein or polypeptide hormones or clotting factors to replace deficient host proteins. Antibodies can be stimulated to human proteins if the deficiency is congenital and immunological tolerance is absent (Parker and Daughaday, 1964) or if there are allotypic differences between the same protein in different human beings. In assays for microbial antigens that circulate over a period of days to many years, such as hepatitis B antigen, masking by complexing with circulating antibody undoubtedly can occur, although it is not yet clear how often it presents a problem or what the most effective solutions are. Antibody formation is also possible to drugs, although interference in immunoassay measurements is unlikely except with drugs that are therapeutically effective at unusually low concentrations in blood. Serum antibodies to digitoxin and morphine have been found in human beings receiving these drugs (Parker, 1974), but only on rare-to-infrequent occasions, and there is no evidence that falsely low or high immunoassay values have resulted.

Goodfriend and his colleagues (1975) have described a plasma protein with high binding affinity ($K_a = 10^6$ to 10^8 liters/mole) for the N-terminal end of desaspartyl angiotensin II (angiotensin II that is missing the aspartyl group at its N-terminal end). It is found in 2% of normals, 6% of unselected hospitalized patients, and 30% of mentally defective individuals maintained in institutions. The protein has very little affinity for undegraded angiotensin II, but it can cause confusion in angiotensin II immunoassays, particularly if the marker is heavily contaminated with desaspartyl angiotensin II, if desaspartyl angiotensin II is formed enzymatically from plasma angiotensin II during extraction, and if the antiangiotensin II antiserum recognizes desaspartyl angiotensin II. Whether the binding protein(s) is a solubilized tissue receptor with unique specificity characteristics, an autoantibody, or a scavenger protein that happens to have binding affinity for desaspartyl angiotensin II remains to be established.

In addition to the various proteins in blood, binding proteins with varying degrees of selectivity for small or large molecular weight ligands are present in many tissues and serve as a potential source of interference in immunological measurements. As a rule, these proteins are inactivated during the initial processing of the tissue, but such inactivation cannot necessarily be assumed.

VALIDATION OF THE IMMUNOASSAY

Because of potential problems in radioimmunoassay measurements in biological samples, each new immunoassay must be systematically validated in the tissue in which it is being utilized. A number of important criteria must be fulfilled before the assay can be applied with an real degree of confidence.

Internal Standards

Tracer quantities of radiolabeled antigen can be added to the sample at the time of initial extraction and used as an internal standard to follow subsequent recovery.* If relatively long (10 to 20 minutes) counting times are used, useful information on recovery can be obtained with as little as 1,000 to 2,000 cpm of tracer. If the tracer is of high specific activity, quantities of tracer on the order of 1 pmole or less provide the needed level of radioactivity. Under these circumstances samples containing added tracer are not substantially changed in their total antigen content, and mixtures of unknown tissue antigen and tracer can be immunoassayed directly. This procedure is of particular value in assays involving elaborate extraction procedures that have variable recoveries. The use of an internal standard is ordinarily feasible even when the radio immunoassay marker and the tracer are labeled with the same radioactive isotope, since the quantity of radioactivity in the tracer is so small. If the required quantity of tracer antigen is too high relative to the antigen present in the tissue, recovery and antigen content can be monitored separately, in simultaneously extracted samples.

---

     * To avoid confusion in subsequent paragraphs, the small quantities of radioactive antigen used to follow recovery during processing will be designated by the term *tracer antigen* or *tracer,* whereas the radioligand molecule in the immunoassay will be termed *immunoassay marker* or *marker.*

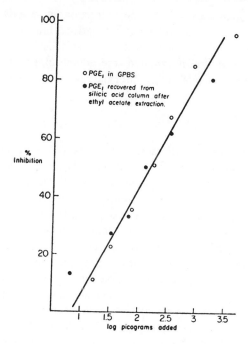

Fig. 9.1. Verification of the PGE radioimmunoassay in serum. PGE_1, 15 to 4,000 pg were added to 1.0 ml of serum, extracted, chromatographed, taken up in buffer, and measured in the PGE radioimmunoassay system. After correcting for recovery (parallel experiments) and subtracting the initial prostaglandin concentration, the data were plotted (closed circles). The calibration curve in buffer (without prior extraction from serum) is plotted for comparison. Note both the linearity of the curve and the close correspondence between the standard curves in extracted and unextracted samples. (Taken from B. M. Jaffe, H. R. Behrman, and C. W. Parker. 1973. J. Clin. Invest. 52:398-405.)

An even more useful form of internal standard is to add larger quantities of unlabeled antigen to tissue samples and see if the expected additivity in the immunoassay is observed (Fig. 9.1). In making this analysis, it is desirable to cover a wide range of added antigen concentrations so that a standard curve can be constructed and compared with the standard curve in buffer. The use of low as well as high concentrations of added antigen is desirable because the sample might contain small quantities of active enzyme with a sufficiently low K_m to be active at low concentrations of antigen. In this case, the enzyme might significantly alter endogenous antigen levels while exerting little or no effect at high total antigen levels. This precaution also applies when metabolic stimulators that produce large rises in tissue-antigen content are used as a means of validating an assay.

As a rule, the internal standard is added during or after tissue extraction is initiated and only provides information on what happens to antigen after the tissue reaction is stopped. In the extraction of blood or other body fluids, it may be useful to add standard antigen immediately before the extraction medium itself. When cells are involved, however, during the time before the extraction is initiated, the added antigen is outside rather than inside the cell and misleading information may be obtained.

More Extensively Purified Samples

Although the advantage of radioimmunoassays lies in their high degree of specificity—ordinarily permitting an analysis to be made on relatively crude tissue extracts—studies of highly purified tissue extracts can be very useful in the initial validation of the assay. If alterations in antigen-marker binding in the immunoassay are indeed a valid measure of the quantity of antigen in the sample, the immunoinhibitory activity should cochromatograph with tracer quantities of labeled antigen, and any losses in activity during processing should be comparable. Since chromatographic systems vary in their discriminatory capacities for different cross-reacting or contaminating antigens, ideally, the analysis should be made in several chromatographic systems. Knowledge of the substances most likely to cross-react in the immunoassay is helpful in determining the most suitable chromatographic systems. Since chromatographic samples usually must be concentrated prior to immunoassay, care is needed to ensure that the antigen is adequately resolubilized after drying and that tracers of chromatographic solvent do not interfere in the assay. This factor can be determined by direct measurements of tracer radioactivity recovery before and after drying and by the inclusion of appropriate solvent blanks.

Proportionality to Quantity of Tissue Extracted
and the Slope of the Tissue Inhibition Curve

Inhibition by antigen in the immunoassay should be proportional to the quantity of tissue extracted (assuming that the analysis is being made in the linear portion of the standard inhibition curve), and the curve obtained by using different quantities of tissue should parallel the standard antigen inhibition curve in buffer. Nonlinearity or nonparallelism may be due to several causes:

1. A diminution in the efficiency with which degradative processes are stopped as the quantity of tissue is increased.
2. Nonlinear effects of degradative enzymes acting later in the extraction process, during storage, or in the assay itself.
3. Nonlinear effects of salts, buffers, alteration in pH, divalent cations,

and contaminants in the distilled water; under these circumstances there is an appreciable blank in the system when buffer alone is extracted and assayed (see below).

4. A carrier effect in which the recovery of antigen is improved as the quantity of antigen processed in increased.

5. The presence of cross-reacting substances in the immunoassay that have a different slope in the dose inhibition curve than the antigen; alternatively, the presence of a contaminating antigen-antibody system (contamination in both the marker and the antibody) for which there is immunoreactivity in the sample.

*Deliberate Destruction of Antigenic Reactivity
by Enzymatic or Chemical Means*

As noted, the antigen may be susceptibe to enzymatic or chemical destruction, which is a possible source of error in immunoassay measurements. On the other hand, when reagents that would be expected to destroy the antigen selectively are added to tissue extracts and the expected fall in immunoreactivity is observed, the result is to help validate the assay. Enzymatic destruction of antigen was used in the initial validation of the cAMP immunoassay. It was possible to show that, in tissue samples treated with cAMP phosphodiesterase, the immunoinhibitory activity in the system was reduced to 10% or less of the original value (Steiner et al., 1969). This finding provided strong evidence that cAMP was indeed what was being measured.

Although enzyme effects on immunoinhibitory activity are very useful in immunoassay validation, the enzyme should be obtainable in a highly purified state, be selective and efficient in its action, and produce a product that does not cross-react immunologically with undegraded antigen. A number of possible sources of misinterpretation should be kept in mind:

1. If the enzyme is not highly purified or if it has a broad substrate specificity, the change in immunoreactivity it produces may involve contaminating or cross-reacting antigens. Nonspecific changes in immunological reactivity involving degradation of interfering macromolecules are also possible.

2. It may be necessary to make additions to the tissue extract to fulfill the divalent cation and pH requirements of the enzyme. Controls are needed to rule out nonspecific effects of these additions in the immunoassay or in reactivating endogenous enzymes specific for other substrates. The longer the time needed to complete the enzymatic destruction of antigen, the greater the likelihood of concurrent changes in cross-reacting or contaminating antigen content.

3. Even if conditions are apparently optimal for enzyme action, unknown inhibitory factors in tissue extracts may prevent the enzymatic reaction from proceeding quantitatively.

4. If the enzyme is not destroyed after it has acted on the tissue antigen, it may act on the immunoassay marker itself, making it appear that immunoinhibitory activity is still present.

In order to avoid some of these problems in interpretation, the digestion can be carried out in the presence of small quantities of radioactive tracer antigen. The reaction mixture is sampled serially and the progress of digestion followed chromatographically as well as immunologically. The fractional loss of immunoinhibitory activity should correspond to the loss observed chromatographically.

Comparisons with Other Assay Methods

When a substance is present in considerable quantity and measurement is possible by a variety of techniques, it is easy to determine whether there is correspondence between immunoassay results and values obtained by other methods. When picomole quantities of antigen must be measured, most analytical techniques lack the needed sensitivity. However, depending on the substance being measured, elegant but tedious analytical methods, such as mass spectroscopy, isotope dilution, or enzyme recycling, can provide valuable reference values. Each has its own pitfalls; and if discrepancies are found, it may be difficult to determine what the true value is. Ideally, as many independent analytical methods as possible should be used in this situation, preferably in the same laboratory, since animal sources and procedural details in handling tissues in different laboratories are important sources of variation and might create the false impression that the methods themselves are producing discrepant results. In addition, exchange of samples or immunoassay reagents between laboratories can also be very helpful in the early phases of assay development.

Parallel bioassay measurements are important in the validation of hormone immunoassays, particularly during the early characterization studies, in order to ensure that what is detected in the immunoassay is largely or entirely the physiologically active protein. Since few bioassays are amenable to precise quantitation and bioassays have major specificity problems of their own, only a gross comparison of activities is possible. However, even relatively imprecise information can be valuable. For example, when bioassay and immunoassay values for LH, HCG, and FSH in urine were compared, a major discrepancy was found. Although the full explanation is not yet clear, there is no doubt that the urine contains altered hormonal molecules (free subunits and variably altered two-chain protein molecules) that differ in immunological and hormonal reactivity from the same gonadotrophins isolated directly from the pituitary or placenta. In LH measurements, the correlation between the immunoassay and the bioassay is improved if urinary rather than pituitary LH is used to prepare the antiserum and as the immunoassay standard (Ryan, 1969).

When initial comparisons between immunoassays and other methods are made and discrepancies are found, it becomes important to screen as many antisera as possible, since some antisera give much closer correlations than others.

Buffer, Tissue, and Stimulatory Agent Blanks

If tissue or plasma that is free of antigen is available, it can be used as a reference standard to determine the tissue blank and to obtain a standard antigen curve in the tissue extract that is not superimposed on the usual baseline tissue antigen level. Hormone-free samples of plasma are sometimes obtainable in endocrine deficiency states, or attempts may be made to remove hormones from plasma by dialysis or by exposure to chaotropic agents, altered conditions of pH and ionic strength, or solid-phase absorbents. Unfortunately, the use of samples from individuals with endocrine deficiency is not completely satisfactory, for it is usually not possible to be certain that an endocrine deficiency is absolute or that immunologically cross-reacting hormones are not present. The hormone-removal approach also leaves much to be desired. The removal of hormones from plasma may be incomplete or may be associated with plasma protein alterations or changes in ionic composition that alter the behavior of the plasma in the immunoassay. The removal of antigen by absorption with antibodies or other high-affinity binding agents attached to a resin is a valuable approach, but spurious results are possible if there is leakage of binding protein from the resin. "Hormone-free" plasma can be obtained from surgically treated animals or from animal species in which the hormone does not cross-react immunologically with the homologous hormone, but the plasma may differ in other respects and misleading results are possible. Thus caution in interpretation is necessary even when the plasma extract is ostensibly antigen free. The problem is much easier when immunoassays for drugs are being validated, since pretreatment serum or plasma can be used as a control (Fig. 9.2).

While it is difficult to obtain a completely satisfactory antigen-free plasma or tissue extract for immunoassay measurements, there is no impediment to ensuring that buffer or stimulatory agents used in experiments with tissue do not produce nonspecific effects. Tubes containing

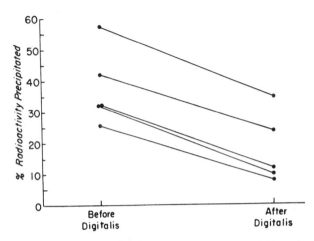

Fig. 9.2. Results from five patients before and after digitalization with digitoxin. Control and postdigitalization sera were compared in the same immunoassay. In every case, postdigitalization sera caused more inhibition of precipitate radioactivity than predigitalization sera (p < 0.001). The variation in predigitalization serum values shown in the graph (from 25 to 60% precipitation of radioactivity) reflects the fact that the immunoassays were carried out at different times under somewhat different conditions. In each instance, other normal sera evaluated at the same time give comparable values. (Taken from G. C. Oliver, B. M. Parker, D. L. Brasfield, and C. W. Parker. 1968. J. Clin. Invest. 47:1035-1042.)

buffer or buffer plus stimulatory agent are set up as blanks and incubated and processed as if tissue were present. After processing, the buffer and reagent extract blanks are evaluated directly for possible effects on radioactive antigen binding or the ability of added unlabeled antigen to inhibit marker binding. Theophylline and norepinephrine are examples of substances that produce unexpected nonspecific immunoassay interference. At high concentrations, both agents inhibit radioactive cGMP binding by antibody even though they do not appear to have structural similarity to cGMP.

Exclusion of Effects of Contaminating
Antigen-Antibody Systems

The preceding discussion assumes that extraneous (*non*immunologically cross-reacting) immune systems are not contributing significantly to overall radioactive antigen binding. This factor is not always easy to establish, since even a highly purified protein can obtain one or more trace contaminants that not only may stimulate an immune response but may also produce a response that is disproportionate to its absolute concentration in the immunizing mixture. Moreover, a contaminant may be labeled more efficiently by ^{125}I than the predominant antigen (Chapter 5), thus creating a situation in which the contaminating immune system contributes significantly to overall radioactive antigen binding. The problem is compounded if the standard antigen solution also contains the contaminant. Useful approaches to this problem include a reevaluation of binding and binding inhibition after further antigen purification and an examination of the inhibitory activity of pure or enriched solutions of suspected contaminants. Since the radioactive antigen is already labeled, only small quantities are needed to study its behavior in suitable chromatographic and radioimmunoelectrophoresis systems, and any new subfractions that are identified can be readily evaluated in the immunoassay.

SUMMARY

1. It cannot be assumed that immunoassay systems that function satisfactorily in buffer necessarily give valid results when blood or tissue is measured.

2. For labile antigens, careful consideration must be given to possible destruction or inactivation of antigen during tissue processing or in the assay itself.

3. Media used in the original tissue incubation or added later during antigen extraction or in the immunoassay itself may introduce acids, bases, inorganic ions, solvents, or solvent residues that interfere in the assay. Effects of such agents can be detected by the use of appropriate buffer and solvent blanks in assay.

4. Depending on the system, endogenous tissue- or plasma-binding proteins that might compete with antibody for antigen may need to be inactivated or removed in order to avoid interference in the immunoassay.

5. Procedures helpful in validating immunoassay results in tissue samples include the use of internal standards, of enzymes to destroy the antigen selectively, comparison of results before and after more extensive antigen purification, comparison of the slope of the antigen inhibition curve with different quantities of tissue to that of standard antigen, and a comparison of the values obtained by immunoassay with those obtained by other methods.

6. The inclusion of radiolabeled antigen as an internal standard at the time of the initial extraction provides valuable information on recovery. It is also a means of establishing that the labeled antigen and the immunoinhibitory activity in the sample behave in the same way chromatographically.

7. The possible presence of contaminating antigen-antibody systems should be carefully considered when an assay is initially validated. This factor is particularly important when the antigen is available in such limited quantities that its purity is uncertain.

Chapter 10

Competitive Assays Utilizing Endogenous Blood or Tissue Receptor Proteins

INTRODUCTION

Although much of the discussion in this monograph and in the literature has centered on assays that utilize antibodies to study competitive binding, the use of endogenous binding proteins for this purpose has almost as long a history.* Plasma proteins with binding affinity for steroid or thyroid hormones have been utilized extensively for competitive binding measurements, beginning with the studies of Ekins (1960) and Murphy et al. (1963). In 1968 Korenman showed that a naturally occurring binding protein extracted from tissue could be used to measure estrogen, and since that time a number of additional assay systems employing tissue-binding proteins have been described. This chapter will consider endogenous receptor assay systems, including certain of their disadvantages and advantages in comparison with radioimmunoassays.

BINDING PROTEINS FROM BLOOD

The blood contains proteins with selective affinity for a variety of circulating hormones. The utilization of these proteins for routine clinical measurements has been studied extensively by Murphy, Ekins, and others (Murphy, 1971; Ekins, 1974). Practical radioreceptor assays have been developed for progesterones, estrogens, androgens, thyroid hormones, corticosteroids, vitamin D derivatives, vitamin B_{12}, and retinal. In general, blood receptor proteins have a somewhat lower overall binding affinity and specificity than tissue receptor proteins or antibodies, although such

---

* For convenience, in our discussion the term *binding protein* or *receptor protein* will be used to describe an endogenous protein with natural affinity for a ligand as distinguished from an antibody, which is always a gamma globulin and must be specifically induced. Of course, strictly speaking, an antibody is also a binding protein.

is not invariably the case. The thyroxin-binding protein present in human serum has a marked degree of specificity for T_4 (Murphy, 1971). The only known examples of cross-reactivity when thyroxin is measured by using this protein are with T_3, D-thyroxine, and diphenylhydantoin, and even these substances cross-react only to a limited extent. Indeed, the binding of T_3 is so low that the protein is unsatisfactory for T_3 measurements.

Several classes of proteins with varying degrees of binding affinity for corticosteroids, estrogens, androgens, and progesterones have been described. There is a corticosteroid-binding globulin (CBG or transcortin) that can be used to measure a variety of corticosteroids in plasma and urine, including cortisol, progesterone, 11-desoxycortisol, desoxycorticosterone, corticosterone, and 17-α-hydroxy-progesterone (Murphy, 1971). Although most applications have utilized human CBG as the binding reagent, it is sometimes advantageous to use dog or monkey CBG. For example, monkey CBG has a relatively high affinity for corticosterone and desoxycorticosterone, and its use results in less interference by cortisol in the assay. Since estrogen treatment markedly increases transcortin concentrations in plasma, plasma from estrogen-treated or pregnant human beings or animals can be used to obtain higher titer-binding protein preparations. Proteins with partial selectivity for progesterone and its congeners can be used when members of the progesterone family are being measured (Murphy, 1971). There is also a relatively specific estrogen-binding protein present in the serum of pregnant rats. Finally, a sex-hormone-binding globulin with selectivity for testosterone, other androgens, estrogen, and 17-B-hydroxysteroids, in general, has been described.

Despite the well-documented usefulness of steroid-binding proteins for routine clinical measurements, most have group rather than specific steroid specificity, and even the group specificity is only partial. Frequently, absolute measurements are possible only after a suitable extraction of chromatographic separation procedure. When the goal is to measure a single substance, this factor is a major disadvantage, although certain of the steroid immunoassays also require that chromatography be done. When the goal is to measure a number of different steroids simultaneously, the lack of specificity may actually be used to advantage, since it is helpful to be able to use the same binding protein to measure a number of different steroids once the chromatographic separation step has been completed. Murphy (1971) has been able to measure eight different steroids by use of CBG.

BINDING PROTEINS FROM TISSUE

Tissue-receptor-binding proteins that have been used in competitive binding assays fall into two major categories, arbitrarily designated in this discussion as type A and type B receptors. Type A receptors are derived from the external cell membrane. Most are receptors for hormones that act at the cell surface to modulate adenylate cyclase activity, including ACTH, glucagon, and growth hormone. The type B receptors are cytoplasmic or nuclear proteins with an affinity for agents that act inside the cell, including cyclic AMP and estrogen.

The estrogen-binding protein first utilized for estrogen assays was obtained from the uterus of pregnant rabbits (Korenman, 1968). It displays considerable specificity for estrogenic steroids. Estradiol, estrone, and estriol all bind to the protein, making it necessary to carry out a preliminary purification step in order to discriminate between these substances.

Cyclic AMP-binding proteins were first described in the adrenal gland in 1969 by Gill and Garren and were later demonstrated in a wide variety of tissues. They were rapidly applied to the measurement of cAMP (Gilman, 1970), and with subsequent refinements less than 0.1 pmole cAMP was reported to be detected by using this method. Practical assays for measuring cAMP have been developed using cAMP-binding proteins from bovine adrenal cortex, bovine skeletal muscle, and calf uterus. These proteins have estimated binding affinities in the 1 to 100×10^7 liters/mole^{-1} range. The applicability of binding proteins from a number of tissues to cAMP measurements is not surprising considering the ability of cAMP to modulate cellular responsiveness in almost every tissue of the body.

Useful binding protein assays have also been developed for human gonadotrophic hormones. In 1972 Lee and Ryan and Catt et al. reported the use of luteinized rat ovaries to develop specific binding assays for human LH and HCG. The binding protein had very little affinity for FSH and prolactin in contrast to the considerable degree of cross-reactivity usually observed with antibodies to LH and HCG. Since the estimated association constants for HCG and LH are as high as 1×10^{10} liters mole^{-1}, sensitivities even higher than in the cAMP-binding protein assay are possible.

Liver, adrenal cortical, and adipose tissue plasma membranes can serve as sources of receptor proteins with high binding affinities for ACTH (Lefkowitz et al., 1970), insulin (Cuatrecasas, 1971), glucagon (Rodbell et al., 1971), and E prostaglandins, although none has been widely applied for routine tissue measurements.

A competitive binding assay utilizing a receptor present in chromatin has been developed to 1-α, 25-dihydroxyvitamin D_3, which is thought to be the active hormonal form of vitamin D (Brumbaugh et al., 1974). The receptor has an affinity for ^3H 1α, 25-dihydroxyvitamin D_3 marker of 1×10^9 liter/mole and is highly specific ($>$ hundredfold higher concentrations of 25-OH vitamin D_3 and vitamin D_3 are needed to produce significant displacement of the marker).

All the preceding tissue receptor proteins are obtained from tissues that respond metabolically in well-defined ways to the hormones in question. Somewhat surprisingly, human lymphocytic cell lines or normal peripheral blood lymphocytes have been reported to contain high-affinity binding sites for HGH (Lesniak et al., 1974) and insulin (Gavin et al., 1972; Gavin et al., 1973) even though clear-cut pharmacologic responses to the two hormones have not been recognized in these cells. It has been suggested that tissues that fail to respond to hormones may still contain adequate numbers of receptors ineffectively coupled to responding enzyme systems. However, a more prosaic explanation is possible, at least for the insulin binding receptor. Since some of the insulin studies were conducted on lymphocyte populations containing 5 to 10% nonlymphocytic cells, some or all of the binding may represent nonspecific uptake of insulin by contaminating phagocytic cells.

Procedural Details in Tissue Receptor, Competitive Binding Assays

The procedures used in competitive binding assays tend to be similar regardless of whether an antibody or a plasma or a tissue-binding protein is involved. A radiolabeled ligand is used, and competitive binding is measured by diminished binding of radiolabel to receptor protein or antibody when inhibitor is present. In binding protein assay systems, optimal conditions for binding vary with the particular protein. Sometimes the assay can be applied directly to crude tissue extracts, but frequently the sample must be partially purified first. When the binding receptor is on the cell surface, the assay may be attempted with intact cells, particularly if a homogenous, easily cultivated cell line is available. But if this is done, consideration should be given to possible variations in receptor number at different stages of the cell cycle. For example, the average number of IgE receptor sites/cell on rat basophilic tumor cells varies, depending on whether cells are harvested during a logarithmic or stationary phase of growth (Isersky et al., 1975).

Relative Advantages of Plasma and Tissue Receptor Competitive Assays as Compared with Radioimmunoassays

Although immunoassays and tissue (or serum-)-binding protein assays may differ significantly in sensitivity or cross-reactivity in a given system, neither method is routinely superior to the other. The two methods suffer from many of the same pitfalls and, by and large, have similar precision and reproducibility. The choice of a method depends on the measurement being made and, to a lesser extent, on whether the investigator is biochemically or immunologically trained. Nonetheless, a few general comments can be made about the relative advantages and disadvantages of the two systems.

Relative Binding Specificity

Depending on the purpose of the assay and what cross-reacting substances may be present in tissue, either a tissue-binding protein assay or a radioimmunoassay may give greater specificity. In cAMP measurements, antibodies can be obtained with very low cross-reactivity with cGMP, whereas considerable cGMP cross-reactivity is present in the binding protein assay system; so from this point of view the immunoassay is preferable. However, since cAMP levels in tissue tend to be considerably higher than cGMP levels, this advantage is not important in most tissues. On the other hand, when HCG or LH is being measured, the appropriate tissue-binding protein normally has much less cross-reactivity for FSH than anti-HCG or anti-LH antibodies do. Extended efforts may lead to the development of antisera with little or no cross-reactivity for FSH, but it may be easier to use a tissue receptor assay from the very beginning. Binding protein assays also present real or theoretical advantages in hormone measurements if biologically inactive hormone fragments that cross-react immunologically with the parent molecule are likely to be present. The result can give the false impression that more physiologically active hormone is present than there actually is. Tissue receptor proteins are unlikely to recognize a hormone that has been degraded to any extent, and this situation will be reflected by both a decreased hormone effect on the tissue and a marked diminution in binding in the radioreceptor assay. Somewhat paradoxically, however, this lack of tolerance to structural alterations in the hormone can be a disadvantage. In the cAMP radioimmunoassay, the antibody readily recognizes 2′0-succinyl derivatives of cAMP, and a phenolic hydroxyl group can be introduced at this position, thus permitting the utilization of ^{125}I as a radioactive marker. This step makes it possible to prepare a radioligand molecule of very high specific activity, thereby creating the potential for exceptionally high sensitivity (see Chapter 5). This same iodinated derivative of cAMP cannot be used in the cAMP-binding protein assay because the reduction in affinity associated with the structural alteration at the 2′0 position is too marked. It is therefore necessary to use a conventional ^{3}H-cAMP marker that is not only less convenient but that also reduces the potential sensitivity of the assay system. In addition, since radioiodination of a hormone inevitably results in structural alterations in the molecule, it may be difficult to obtain a high degree of binding with radioiodinated hormones in a tissue receptor assay. For example, in radioreceptor assays for ACTH, a major portion of the iodinated ACTH fails to react with the receptor protein even though the ^{125}I ACTH has been purified after iodination and, by ordinary chromatographic and immunological criteria, appears to be undamaged (Odell et al., 1971). Although satisfactory sensitivity may still be obtainable, the practical range over which inhibition of binding can be measured is considerable reduced. Moreover, in tissue receptor assays, increased difficulty would be anticipated in attempting to use a radioiodinating antigen over an extended period of time. Thus the inherent problems associated with radioiodination of polypeptide or protein hormones are likely to be magnified when tissue receptor assays are used.

There are other potential problems in tissue receptor assays. The binding affinities of a tissue protein may be subject to allosteric modulation by substances in the tissue sample, thus creating a potential source of interference in the assay. For example, the binding of HCG by its receptor protein in bovine corpus luteum cell membranes is substantially reduced at high adenine, guanine, and cytosine nucleotide concentrations (Rao, 1974). GTP exerts a similar effect on the binding of glucagon to its receptor in liver membranes (Rodbell et al., 1971). These inhibitory effects appear to involve nucleotide-binding sites outside the hormone-binding region and are noncompetitive in nature. Allosteric effects on binding should not be a problem in radioimmunoassays with the possible exception of assays involving unheated serum samples, where effects of complement on binding would need to be considered.

Nonspecific binding can also present problems in binding protein assays, as is evident in studies with catecholamine receptor proteins, where what initially appeared to be specific catecholamine receptors failed to exhibit the expected degree of stereospecificity in their binding. Although all tissues that respond to catecholamines undoubtedly contain specific catecholamine receptors, as a rule, they are masked by tissue constituents that bind catecholamines nonselectively and have a much greater overall catecholamine-binding capacity. Under these circumstances it is not possible to develop a truly specific or sensitive assay, although eventually it may be possible to do so by better tissue selection or more intensive purification of the receptor. Indeed, some improvement in binding specificity has already been obtained by using avian erythrocyte membranes as a source of catecholamine receptors. Nonspecific binding problems tend to be minimal or absent with antibodies; and if they exist at all, they can be further reduced by the use of purified gamma globulin fractions or specifically purified antibodies.

Binding Affinity and Sensitivity

The range in binding affinities of antibodies and receptor-binding proteins assays overlaps to a large extent. For example, the equilibrium constants of tissue receptor proteins for HCG, insulin, and glucagon are in the range of 10^8 to 10^{11} liters/mole; for properly selected antibody to the same proteins, the operational affinity (avidity) is in the 10^{10} to 10^{13} liters/mole range. Both assay methods should therefore permit sensitivities in the low picomole-to-low femtomole range. Radioimmunoassay and tissue receptor protein assays for cAMP are comparable in sensitivity (0.2 to 2.0 pmoles), although with the best anti-cAMP antisera, the immunoassay is probably at least severalfold more sensitive (sensitivities in the 20 to 50 femtomole range).* Neither assay system operates at its maximal sensitivity unless interfering substances and any variation introduced during the tissue extraction are kept to a minimum. When the cAMP in tissue samples is converted to 2'0-succinyl cAMP by reaction with succinic anhydride, the sensitivity of the cAMP immunoassay system is increased by 2 to 3 orders of magnitude to sensitivities below 1 femtomole, making it much more sensitive than binding protein assay (the comparison is made on unsuccinylated samples, since succinylation is undersirable in the binding protein assay). In measurement of cGMP, the immunoassay is much more sensitive than existing tissue receptor assays even in unsuccinylated samples.

Serum-receptor protein assay systems tend to have considerably lower sensitivities than the corresponding immunoassays, but since high sensitivity may not be needed, this is not necessarily an important advantage.

---

* It is often difficult to compare reported sensitivities from different laboratories. Obviously the practical sensitivity of an assay system is the sensitivity obtainable in tissue extracts. The apparent sensitivity of a system can be manipulated to some extent by use of nonequilibrium assay conditions, unusually small incubation volumes, or long counting times. Although, in theory, samples can be always concentrated into small volumes, this process may result in an unacceptable increase in nonspecific interference in the assay unless the samples are chromatographed, and the chromatography procedure itself may increase intra-assay variability. In addition, investigators vary in what they are willing to accept as a "significant" diminution in binding in the low dose end of the standard inhibition curve.

Problems in Assay Development

UTILIZATION OF A PREVIOUSLY DESCRIBED ASSAY

In general, once a suitable tissue-binding protein assay system has been described, it should be possible for other laboratories to work with the same animal species, identify and isolate the protein, and obtain an identical binding system. In addition, the binding protein should theoretically exhibit homogeneous binding to ligand. This situation is not true for radioimmunoassays, where individual antisera vary to some extent in their specificity and affinity characteristics and are likely to exhibit heterogeneous binding. Nonetheless, it certainly cannot be assumed that all tissue receptor assays will be free of interlaboratory variation. Hormone receptors in liver can vary in their concentration or affinity, depending on the physiological status of the animal, with particularly marked effects being seen following adrenalectomy or hypothesectomy. Other potential sources of variation are the strain or nutritional status of the animal. Even assuming that the tissue available for extraction is, in fact, similar or identical in its binding characteristics to that used by other investigators, the tissue concentrations of most of these proteins are low, and they are frequently less easily obtainable in sizable quantities than antibodies and naturally occurring serum-binding proteins. In addition, depending on their location in the cell, they may be difficult to extract in a soluble form, particularly if the protein is derived from the plasma membrane. While some binding proteins are stable and easy to obtain in a usable state, others present major preparative problems. Therefore reproducible preparations may be difficult to obtain, even within the same laboratory, to say nothing of the problems that can arise when other laboratories attempt to utilize the same procedure. Moreover, originally satisfactory tissue-binding preparations may prove to be quite unstable despite being stored under apparently optimal conditions. Instability may even be a problem during performance of the binding assay itself. Considering these potential difficulties, the theoretical possibility of being able to utilize a tissue receptor protein identical to that in other laboratories may not be readily realized in practice, or even if it is, the practical advantage of having such a protein may turn out to be more imagined than real. If an assay is going to be needed over a period of many months to years, the investment of the time needed to obtain a suitable antiserum may well be worth the effort. In addition, many commonly used antisera are now available commercially.

DEVELOPMENT OF NEW ASSAYS

Workable radioimmunoassays have been obtained to such a large number of substances of differing molecular properties that it can be assumed that new assays will be achievable with all except the smallest or most unstable molecules. A number of factors make it unlikely that this degree of flexibility will be achievable in tissue receptor systems:

1. Drugs and even many normal tissue constituents may not be bound with sufficient affinity by endogenous macromolecules to permit the development of practical competitive binding assays. Although extensive screening studies in microorganisms and plants may eventually unearth some presently unidentified binding proteins, the greatest new source of binding reagents, apart from any new antibodies that may be developed, may come from more sophisticated techniques of organic synthesis (e.g., by de novo synthesis of macromolecules with selective binding properties).

2. Even though a number of additional tissue or serum receptor proteins might theoretically be explored for assay development, because of problems of receptor instability or insolubility discussed earlier, some easily demonstrated tissue receptor proteins may not be suitable for radioreceptor assay use. For example, extensive attempts to develop receptor assays for aldosterone in tissues responding to this agent have met with very limited success. Moreover, certain of the type-B tissue receptor proteins recognize the metabolically altered hormone rather than the form of the hormone that circulates in plasma and so are not suitable for plasma measurements. For example, although tissue receptors specific for members of the testosterone series exist, they appear to have primary specificity for 5-α-dihydrotestosterone, a metabolic conversion product of testosterone formed in the tissue, rather than testosterone itself (Korenman and Sanborn, 1971). Thus even when a tissue is highly responsive biochemically and appears to bind a hormone with a high degree of affinity, the success of the tissue-receptor protein approach is unpredictable.

SUMMARY

1. Endogenous blood or tissue-receptor-binding proteins are alternative reagents to antibodies in the development of sensitive competitive binding assays. Receptor protein assays are similar to radioimmunoassays in the use of competitive decreases in radioactive ligand binding as a measure of unlabeled ligand concentration. They suffer from many of the same pitfalls and generally are similar in precision and reproducibility.

2. Using binding proteins present in blood, practical assays for T$_4$,

vitamin B_{12}, and a wide variety of corticosteroids and sex hormones have been developed. Using proteins present in tissue, sensitive methods for measuring cAMP, LH, HCG, ACTH, glucagon, insulin, prostaglandin E_1,1-α-25-dihydroxyvitamin D_3, and growth hormone are available, although only a portion is in everyday use for tissue measurements.

3. The likelihood that a tissue might contain a protein suitable for use in a radioreceptor assay can normally be predicted from the way it responds biochemically. However, not all receptor proteins lend themselves to the development of practical assays, particularly proteins derived from particulate subcellular fractions.

4. Tissue receptor proteins are less likely to bind to partially damaged or fragmented protein than antibody, which is a mixed blessing in that it reduces the likelihood that biologically inactive protein fragments would be measured but also increases the susceptibility of the assay to nonspecific changes in marker binding as a result of the radiolabeling itself. Diminished binding following the introduction of radioiodine is even more marked in the cAMP-binding protein assay and a ^{3}H marker must be used—in contrast to the cAMP radioimmunoassay, where an iodinated cAMP marker can be prepared and shown to bind with high affinity to antibody.

Chapter 11

Possible Practical Approaches to Problems
of Antigenic Cross-reactivity

INTRODUCTION

The subject of antigenic cross-reactivity has been developed in some detail in preceding chapters. Although cross-reactivity may present few if any difficulties, it is a major source of misinterpretation in some systems. Thus it is useful at this point to recapitulate the general types of antigenic cross-reactivity and consider possible practical solutions.

The different kinds of immunologic cross-reactivity fall into three major categories. One type is represented by two proteins, one with determinants AB and the second with the identical determinant A and an unrelated determinant C.* In this case, an antibody directed solely toward B should detect protein AB in the presence of AC with no demonstrable cross-reactivity. The problem, then, is to obtain an effective anti-B antiserum, not contaminated by anti-A antibody. The second type of cross-reactivity is illustrated by two proteins, AB and A′C. Here the only determinants that resemble one another are structurally similar but not identical. A third type of cross-reactivity is exhibited by proteins A-B and A′-B or A-B′. In this case, it may be difficult or impossible to obtain a completely specific antiserum, although the inherent cross-reactivity between A and A′ or B and B′ may be reduced to a minimum by the proper selection of an antiserum.

The problem of binding cross-reactivity can be handled by eliminating the antibody altogether and replacing it with a tissue-binding protein (which may, however, have cross-reactivity problems of its own; Chapter 10) or by appropriate manipulations within the immunoassay system itself. The ensuing discussion will deal with the second approach.

---

* For purposes of discussion, the possibility that there might be multiple As, Bs, and Cs will be ignored.

190

SPECIFIC APPROACHES TO PROBLEMS OF IMMUNOLOGICAL CROSS-REACTIVITY

Attempts to minimize antigenic cross-reactivity may be exerted at any one (or more) of four stages of immunoassay development:

1. At the time of the immunization (by altering the immunizing antigen or immunization conditions).

2. At the time that the antiserum is obtained (by partial purification to eliminate cross-reacting antibodies or careful screening to select the most specific antisera).

3. At the time that the tissue is extracted in preparation for assay (by utilizing separation procedures that eliminate the cross-reacting antigen or by chemical modification of the antigen mixture to alter the relative reactivities of the homologous and cross-reacting antigens with antibody).

4. At the time of the assay itself (by utilizing a radioindicator molecule that is devoid of the cross-reacting determinants, by assaying in the presence of excess cross-reacting antigen, or by carrying out simultaneous assays for the homologous and cross-reacting antigens).

Each of these approaches will now be discussed in greater detail.

Immunization Methods Designed to Minimize Problems of Immunologic Cross-reactivity

IMMUNIZATION OF MULTIPLE ANIMALS AND MULTIPLE ANIMAL SPECIES

Animals vary in the areas on antigen molecule that they recognize as foreign, even within the same species, which can be an important factor in immunologic cross-reactivity. Thus in the first example cited earlier, in which protein AB cross-reacts with protein AC, by immunizing enough animals with AB and utilizing one or several animal species, it may be possible to find an animal that responds well to determinant B and poorly to determinant A. The variable cross-reactivity in different anti-cAMP antisera is illustrated in Table 11.1. Since antiserum specificity may vary with time during immunization, it is desirable often to examine antisera repeatedly during the immunization process in order to maximize specificity.

IMMUNIZATION WITH ANTIGEN FRAGMENTS

If the structure of the antigen is favorable, it may be possible to remove A from B by enzymatic or chemical proteolysis and immunize with frag-

Table 11.1

Sensitivity and specificity of various anti-cAMP antibodies.

Antisera	Maximal sensitivity		Relative binding affinity	
	Serum dilution	cAMP (pmoles/tube)	ATP (%)	cGMP (%)
RC A-1	1:5,000	1	0.002	0.01
RC A-3	1:5,000	1	0.0001	0.005
RC A-7	1:5,000	0.25	0.002	0.01
SM-381	1:5,000	0.025	0.00001	0.01
SM-291	1:4,000	0.05	0.01	0.10
LCA-1	1:40,000	0.25	0.0001	1.0
LCA-2	1:40,000	0.25	0.0001	1.0

Sensitivity values are based on the minimal concentration of cAMP that causes linear displacement in the immunoassay. Cross-reactivity values are based on the minimal quantity of inhibitor required to produce displacement of marker comparable to that of cAMP. All the antisera were from rabbits immunized with 2'0-succinyl cAMP albumin. (Taken from Steiner, 1974, Table I.)

ments containing only B. This process is more easily accomplished with some proteins than others. For example, immunoglobulins and hormones, such as LH and HCG, are readily separated into independent antigenic domains that retain their immunizing capacity, thus permitting the generation of more specific antisera (Fig. 11.1); the approach is much less successful with serum albumins. If antigen fragments are used for immunization, they must be carefully purified, since even small quantities of contaminating intact protein may give rise to significant amounts of cross-reacting antibody.

USE OF CONJUGATION PROCEDURES TO DIRECT THE
IMMUNE RESPONSE TO STRUCTURALLY UNIQUE OR MINIMALLY
CROSS-REACTIVE AREAS OF THE MOLECULE

In immunizing with small molecular weight polypeptides, where conjugation to protein is normally the procedure of choice, one can conjugate the peptide to proteins through the region most likely to cross-react immunologically. Under favorable circumstances this step will help direct the response to structurally distinguishable areas in the peptide. Thus in the case of an oligopeptide containing cross-reacting determinant A and non-cross-reacting determinant B, the idea would be to conjugate the polypeptide through A, favoring the formation of antibodies directed primarily toward B. (See Fig. 2.2, Chapter 2.) In principle, this approach is also applicable to proteins if the chemical reactivity of unwanted determinant

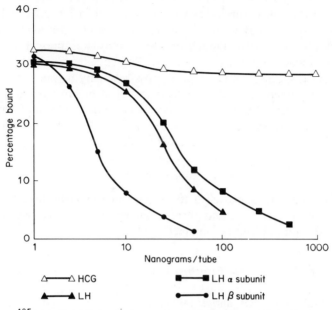

Fig. 11.1. Inhibition of binding of labeled luteinizing hormone (LH) β subunit to an antiserum prepared against LHβ subunit by human chorionic gonadotrophin (HCG), LH, αLH subunit (purified LH α chain) and βLH subunit (purified LH β chain). (Taken from H. S. Jacobs, and N. F. Lawton. 1974. Brit. Med. Bull. 30:55-61.)

A is such that it can be selectively masked or otherwise altered so as to diminish the response to A. Immunization with A-B complexed with anti-A antibodies is another way in which the formation of anti-A antibodies might be minimized.

USE OF A THIRD CROSS-REACTING PROTEIN FOR IMMUNIZATION

If immunization with A-B produces too much immunologic cross-reactivity, it may be possible to obtain the same protein from another species and obtain antibodies with less marked cross-reactivity. Theoretically, it is possible if the new protein is B-D, B'-D, A'-B, or even A'-B' (if A' is poorly immunogenic or differs more from A than B' does from B). The approach was utilized empirically by Midgley et al. (1971) and Hendrick et al. (1971) to reduce immunologic cross-reactivity between

FSH, LH, and TSH, which have similar α chains but different β chains. They found that when antibodies were prepared to ovine FSH and human FSH was used as a marker, little or no cross-reactivity with human LH and TSH was observed [even though cross-reactivity was present in the homologous (ovine FSH marker) system]. Subsequent studies showed that, within a given species, immunological cross-reactivity between the different hormones is conferred by the α chain; this type of cross-reactivity drops out when a species barrier is crossed. Nonetheless, adequate binding is obtained in the heterologous system because the β chains of FSH exhibit considerable interspecies cross-reactivity (Vaitukaitis et al., 1972).

BY IMMUNIZATION OF PARTIALLY TOLERANT ANIMALS

Another possible approach is to produce immunologic tolerance to the cross-reacting protein AC and then immunize with AB in the hope that only anti-B antibody will be obtained.

Absorption to Eliminate the Cross-reacting Antibody

If available anti-AB antisera have been screened and all are cross-reactive with protein A-C, it may be possible to improve their specificity by removing or blocking the anti-A antibody (Fig. 11.2). Ideally, the process is accomplished by use of a solid-phase immunoabsorbent containing the A determinant, which ensures that the anti-A antibody is removed entirely from the system. The protein AC (or a suitable fragment derived from AB containing only the A fragment) is covalently attached to a solid matrix, such as Sepharose, usually with cyanogen bromide or bromoacetyl bromide, and used to absorb the antiserum or gamma globulin fraction. As a rule, the absorption is carried out at 4°C by passing the antiserum over several fresh batches of immunoabsorbent. If complete removal of anti-A antibody seems desirable, it may be necessary to absorb the antiserum repeatedly with a large excess of insolubilized A-C. In this case, it is important to be certain that A-C is entirely free of A-B. Once the absorption is completed, samples from each stage of the process are monitored for cross-reactivity in the immunoassay.

In practice, the removal of contaminating antibodies by solid-phase absorption generally works well, and the method is a valuable one for improving the specificity of an antiserum. However, some care is needed to ensure that the insolubilized antigen does not leak from the absorbent into the serum, for leakage might create problems in interpretation in the immunoassay.

Purification by absorption to insolubilized B, followed by recovery of

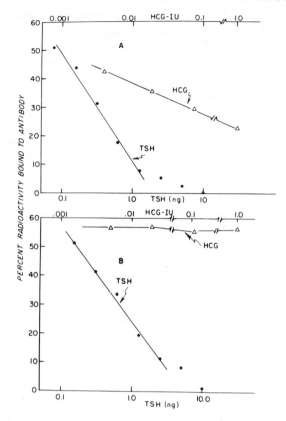

Fig. 11.2. The effect of human chorionic gonadotropin (HCG) on the binding of labeled TSH by anti-TSH serum (a) Untreated anti-TSH serum. (b) Anti-TSH serum previously absorbed with HCG. (Taken from R. D. Utiger. 1965. *In* C. Cassaro, and M. Andreoli (Eds.). Current topics in thyroid research. Academic Press, New York. pp. 513–526.)

anti-B antibody by specific or nonspecific elution, may also be attempted (see Chapter 6).

Partial Purification or Chemical Modification
of the Tissue Sample

ELIMINATION OR SELECTIVE DESTRUCTION OF
HOMOLOGOUS OR CROSS-REACTING ANTIGEN

If either A-B or A-C (but not both) is highly susceptible to selective enzymatic or chemical degradation, then the destructive reaction can be used to help estimate the relative amounts of A-B and A-C. If A-B can be selectively destroyed, any residual immunological reactivity will be due to A-C, and A-B can be determined by difference. If A-C can be selectively destroyed, assays for A-B can be conducted routinely in A-C free samples. Alternatively, it may be possible to remove AC by using a suitable chromatographic separation. This step is particularly valuable when more than two immunologically cross-reacting antigens are present. For example, in the immunoassay of prostaglandins in serum or plasma, at least three major prostaglandin groups are present (PGA, PGF, and PGE), all of which could contain as many as three individual members and which cross-react with one another (Fig. 11.3). In addition, there are the various pros-

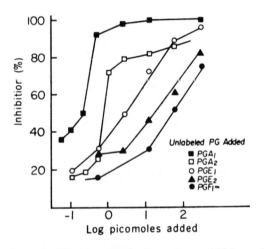

Fig. 11.3. Cross-reactions of different prostaglandins using anti-PGA$_1$ antibody and PGE$_1$ marker. (Taken from B. M. Jaffe, J. W. Smith, W. T. Newton, and C. W. Parker. 1971. Science. 171:494-496.)

taglandin peroxides and precursors, as well as biologically inactive prostaglandin degradation products, all of which cross-react in the assay. Even if antisera and radioimmunoassay markers were available for every possible antigenic species, unless the general level of antigenic cross-reactivity were very low, it would be difficult to be certain of the absolute quantities of each. Therefore at least one preliminary chromatographic separation step is highly desirable. Fortunately, prostaglandin groups can be clearly separated (Fig. 11.4). For the same reason, chromatographic separation may also be desirable with steroid hormones, extensively metabolized drugs, or polypeptide hormones that circulate in multiple molecular forms (see also Chapter 12).

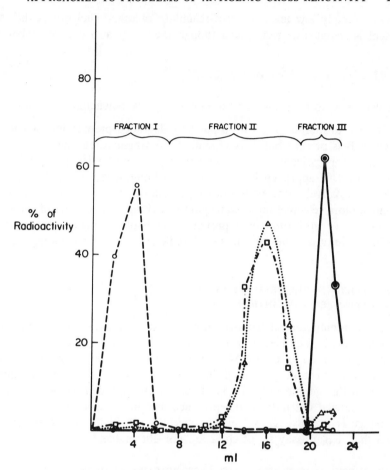

Fig. 11.4. Separation of prostaglandin groups by silicic acid chromatography; [^{3}H] PGA$_1$ 100,000 cpm (open circles), [^{3}H] PGE$_1$ 100,000 cpm (open squares), or [^{3}H] PGF$_{1\alpha}$ 60,000 cpm (closed circles) was added to serum and extracted. After evaporation of the organic phase, samples were chromatographed on silicic acid columns, concentrated, and counted. For comparison, [^{3}H] PGE$_1$ was chromatographed without prior extraction from serum (open triangles). Note the virtually complete separation of prostaglandin groups obtained. (Taken from B. M. Jaffe, H. R. Behrman, and C. W. Parker. 1973. J. Clin. Invest. 52:398-405.)

CHEMICAL MODIFICATION OF THE ANTIGEN MIXTURE

As noted earlier (Chapters 2 and 6), when conventional anti-cAMP antibodies are used, the binding affinity is much greater for 2'0-succinyl-cAMP than for cAMP itself (Fig. 6.1). If tissue samples containing cAMP are succinylated, the sensitivity of the assay for cAMP is not only increased but the already low level of cross-reactivity of other nucleotides that are present is reduced as well (even though they may also be succinylated).

Modifications at the Time of the Assay

THE USE OF A NON-CROSS-REACTING RADIOINDICATOR MOLECULE

Instead of immunizing with a partially degraded preparation of antigen in which B is present but A is absent, the B fragment can be used as the radioindicator molecule, bypassing any anti-A antibodies present in the antiserum. This approach has been used in immunoassays for ACTH and PTH. Alternatively, one of the other procedures described earlier for obtaining a more selective immune response, such as chemical modification of the antigen or utilization of a protein from another species, can be employed to improve the specificity of radioactive antigen binding in the assay.

MEASUREMENT IN THE PRESENCE OF EXCESS CROSS-REACTING ANTIGEN

If the immunological cross-reactivity of AC is weak, then AC may only partially inhibit radioactive antigen binding, even at high concentrations. In this situation an excess of AC can be added to the tissue sample, damping out the effect of the small but variable amounts of AC originally present in the sample (Fig. 11.5). If an excess is added, standard curves must be carried out both in the presence and the absence of AC. A disadvantage is that excess AC may reduce the sensitivity of the system so much that useful assay sensitivities are not obtainable.

SIMULTANEOUS IMMUNOASSAYS FOR CROSS-REACTING ANTIGENS

If anti-AC antibody and radioiodinated AC antigen are available, tissue samples can be assayed in parallel in the AC and the AB systems. On the basis of the standard curves for AC and AB in each of the two systems and the use of simultaneous equations, it should be possible to arrive at the approximate contributions of AB and AC in each system.

REFINEMENT OF THE ASSAY CONDITIONS

The conditions of the immunoassay itself, the degree of nonspecific damage to antigenic reactivity of the marker, the quantity of antibody used, and even the portion of the antigen-binding curve utilized in the assay may all influence the degree of cross-reactivity seen in the immunoassay. For example, reference has already been made to the effect of pH on antigenic

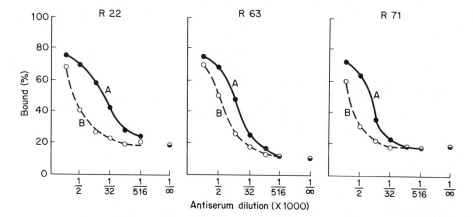

Fig. 11.5. Use of paired antiserum dilution curves to screen antisera for cross-reactivity. R22, R63, and R71 are anti-FSH sera. The A curves contain ^{125}I-FSH 1.0 ng/ml and anti-FSH antibody only. The B curves also contain 9.0 ng/ml unlabeled FSH. All tubes contain LH 100 ng/ml. The separation of the A and B curves indicates the antiserum's ability to detect different concentrations of the specific antigen (FSH) in the presence of an excess of a cross-reacting substance (LH). Antiserum R22 is seen to be superior in this respect. (Taken from W. M. Hunter. 1973. *In* D. M. Weir (Ed.). Handbook of experimental immunology. Blackwell Scientific Publications, Oxford. pp. 17.1–17.36.)

cross-reactivity when human PTH is measured by radioimmunoassay (Fischer et al., 1974).

SUMMARY

1. Attempts to minimize assay cross-reactivity may be exerted at any of four stages of immunoassay development: (a) at the time of immunization (by immunizing multiple animals and animal species, by use of a fragmented, selectively conjugated, chemically modified, or cross-reacting antigen, or by use of partially tolerant animals); (b) at the time that the antibody is obtained (by careful antiserum selection or by partial purification or absorption of an antiserum); (c) at the time that the tissue extract is prepared for assay (by partial purification or selective chemical modification of the antigen); (d) at the time of the immunoassay itself (by use of radiolabeled ligand that is free of cross-reacting determinants, by assaying in cross-reacting antigen excess, by carrying out simultaneous immunoassays for homologous and cross-reacting antigens, or simply by a detailed analysis of optimal assay conditions).

2. If the problem of cross-reactivity is difficult to eliminate, the use of a tissue-receptor protein assay (see Chapter 10) may be worth considering.

Chapter 12

Limitations or Disadvantages of
Radioimmunoassays

Radioimmunoassays offer many advantages in terms of sensitivity, specificity, and convenience, but they also have inherent limitations and disadvantages. Some of the limitations are unique or largely restricted to immunoassays; other represent more general problems in interpretation that arise when quantitative measurements in blood, urine, or tissue are used as an index of what the pharmacologic or physiologic response might be in the organism as a whole.

Possible Problems in Interpretation
When Overall Antigen Reactivity is Measured

Under ideal circumstances the antigen would be a single molecular species with no possibility of interference by cross-reacting antigens. However, such is rarely if ever the case.

1. Hormones tend to occur in families with partial structural homology between individual members of the same family (e.g., ACTH, α- and β-MSH; FSH, LH, HCG, and TSH; GH and prolactin). As a result, hormone measurements are normally being made in the presence of potentially cross-reacting antigens.

2. Individual hormones may circulate in several molecular forms that vary in their biological and immunological reactivity (e.g., ordinary insulin, "big" insulin, and partially degraded insulin).

3. Many drugs are partially degraded to a large number of new products that differ from the parent drug in their pharmacologic and antigenic reactivity.

Once cross-reacting antigens have been identified, they can be studied for their apparent contribution to overall antigenic reactivity when an average tissue sample is measured. However, even assuming that this contribution is small, the possibility that rare tissue samples might contain unexpectedly high levels of cross-reacting antigen must be considered. In this event, inhibition produced by cross-reacting antigen would be superimposed on that of the homologous antigen, and a falsely high estimate of homologous antigen content would be obtained. The true situation would only become evident if the samples were studied in greater detail. Fortunately, problems of this kind are unusual and can sometimes be anticipated from a knowledge of clinical situations (e.g., pregnancy) in which unusually high levels of cross-reacting antigens occur.

UNEXPECTED CROSS-REACTIONS

An assay may have been in use for some time before unexpected sources of false positives or immunologic cross-reactivity are observed. A case in point is the positive urine test for morphine in individuals ingesting bread or coffeecake that contains poppy seeds (Sunshine, 1974). The potential problems arising from cross-reactions of this kind in screening studies for morphine addicts are obvious, and it need hardly be emphasized that positive results by immunoassay should be verified by an independent method. Despite the problem of cross-reactivity, the rapidity of immunological techniques for detecting morphine and its congeners makes them valuable for initial screening. While unexpected cross-reactions may be recognized only after an assay has been in use for some time, the studies of Adler and his colleagues (1972), in which a large group of hospitalized patients taking a variety of drugs that might cross-react with morphine were screened in the morphine hemagglutination inhibition assay, provide a useful model for the type of study that may lead to earlier recognition of unexpected cross-reactions.

INHERENT PITFALLS AND INACCURACIES APART FROM ANTIGEN CROSS-REACTIVITY PER SE

The many pitfalls in immunoassay measurements, including insufficiently rapid tissue processing, failure to inactivate degradative enzymes, salt and pH effects, and improper sample storage, are discussed in detail in Chapter 9.

LACK OF CLOSE CORRELATION BETWEEN ABSOLUTE BLOOD OR TISSUE LEVELS AND THE PHARMACOLOGIC OR TOXIC RESPONSE

The value of measuring blood drug levels has now been established in a number of clinical settings:

1. In monitoring routine drug therapy with digitoxin, digoxin, theophylline, salicylates, dilantin, autonomic blocking agents, and hydralazine.

2. In known or suspected acute drug poisoning, especially if phenobarbital, barbital, salicylate, iron, lithium, opiate, paracetamol, or digitalis is a possible agent (Prescott, 1974).

3. In planning further therapy following hemodialysis or in association with severe renal, liver, or gastrointestinal disease, where the metabolism or excretion of a drug may be markedly altered.

This list will undoubtedly continue to expand as additional methods for measuring drugs are developed. However, as in any other clinical laboratory measurement, there is the danger that the physician will rely exclusively on the drug level, ignoring how and when the sample was drawn, how much drug was taken, and even time-honored clinical signs of toxicity. Serious problems in interpretation are possible in a number of situations:

1. Some drugs are concentrated in tissue to a major extent, and blood levels can never be a really useful index of the total quantity of effective drug in the body.

2. Many drugs are extensively bound to serum proteins, and the total concentrations of the drug in blood may be an inexact measure of the quantity of drug immediately available to tissue. Problems in interpretations are compounded if drugs that might compete for the same binding sites on serum proteins are being administered simultaneously or if hypoproteinemia is present. In addition, in individuals receiving animal or human hormone replacement therapy [e.g., bovine insulin (Yalow and Berson, 1971) or human growth hormone (Parker and Daughaday, 1964)], antibody induction may occur, leading to the formation of circulating antigen-antibody complexes. Depending on the class of antibody and the molecular structure of the antigen, antigen molecules already complexed to human antibody may or may not be biologically active and may or may not be detected by the animal antiserum used in the immunoassay. Complexing of circulating antigen by endogenous antibody is also possible in viremic states and can explain a portion of the negative immunoassays for hepatitis B antigen in individuals infected with this agent (Aach et al., 1973).

3. A number of drugs vary in their effectiveness, depending on pH or electrolyte concentrations in blood and tissues. For example, the effects of digitalis on cardiac tissue are exaggerated when either hypokalemia or hypercalcemia is present. In addition, hypoxia, hyperthyroidism, underlying myocardial disease, and concurrent drug therapy may all influence the likelihood of digitalis-induced cardiac toxicity. Of course, digitalis immunoassays are of great diagnostic value in selected individuals (see Fig. 12.1), particularly those with acute congestive heart failure or

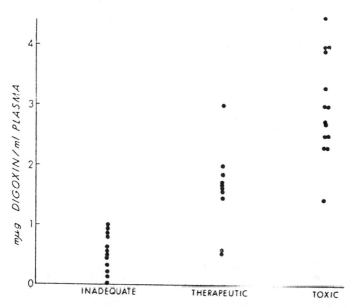

Fig. 12.1. Plasma digoxin levels as determined by radioimmunoassay in individuals judged clinically inadequately digitalized, adequately digitalized, or toxic. Despite some overlap, a highly significant difference was found between inadequately and adequately digitalized patients ($p < 0.001$) and adequately digitalized and toxic patients ($p < 0.001$). (Taken from G. C. Oliver, B. M. Parker, and C. W. Parker. 1971. Amer. J. Med. 51:186-192.)

cardiac arrhythmias, where a decision as to whether to give more drug or withhold the drug may be difficult on clinical grounds alone. Nonetheless, when blood levels are obtained, they must be interpreted in the context of the therapeutic situation at hand, taking into account all other information available on possible toxic effects of the drug.

4. Depending on the drug, blood levels may be importantly influenced by whether the blood is allowed to hemolyze or by when it is drawn relative to the preceding dose (Fig. 12.2). In addition, many hormones exhibit significant diurnal variation, and the time at which blood samples are taken for hormone measurements must be given careful consideration.

5. If prevention of drug toxicity is the goal, it must be recognized that many examples are known in which there is no direct relationship between drug dosage and toxicity.

6. A number of commonly used drugs are therapeutically active only after metabolic conversion in tissue (e.g., cyclophosphamide). In this case, it may be more useful to measure the metabolite than the drug itself.

Thus even assuming that drug levels can be measured and that the values are accurate, a false sense of security in regard to the value of the information obtained must be avoided.

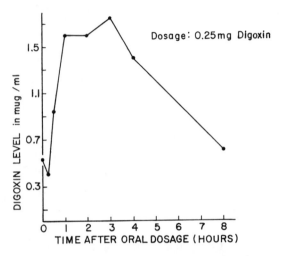

Fig. 12.2. Effect of time of collection of sample in relation to previous dose on measured digoxin levels in plasma. Following oral ingestion of a 0.25-mg digoxin tablet, there was a prompt rise in plasma digoxin concentration. This peak concentration occurred sometime between 1 and 4 hours, following which there was a fairly rapid fall in concentration. From 8 hours to 24 hours, there was a further slight fall. (Taken from G. C. Oliver, B. M. Parker, and C. W. Parker. 1971. Amer. J. Med. 51:186-192.)

SPECIAL PROBLEMS WITH IMMUNOASSAYS THAT ARE IN INFREQUENT USE

With the increasing popularity of immunoassays, commercial immunoassay reagents or reagent kits have become available for a variety of pharmacologic hormonal and biochemical measurements. Many of these commercial reagents are relatively expensive, but sometimes it is more worthwhile to buy ready-made reagents than to invest the time and effort needed to generate and characterize one's own antisera. Needless to say, commercial antisera do not always live up to advanced billing in terms of sensitivity or specificity. Even assuming that a reliable supplier can be identified, it is important to monitor for possible deterioration of immunoassay reagents with continued use or storage. Since seasoned laboratories using immunoassays on a day-by-day basis experience sporadic and apparently unexplained difficulties in assay sensitivity or reproducibility, it is certain that purchasers of immunoassay reagents will encounter many of the same problems. The problem may be compounded if an immunoassay is used on an infrequent or irregular basis. In addition, if the sample load is small, immunoassay methods become relatively inefficient. One of the main advantages of immunoassays is their applicability to the rapid processing of many samples, but regardless of how few samples are measured, it is still necessary to include a full standard curve and antigen and antibody controls in each assay. Thus if measurements are being made infrequently, other methods may be far more preferable, particularly if inexpensive chemical assay methods with the needed degree of sensitivity and reproducibility are available.

FUNCTIONALLY INACTIVE PROTEINS THAT RETAIN THEIR FULL ANTIGENIC REACTIVITY

There are a number of well-studied examples in the complement and clotting literature in which a functionally inactive plasma protein retains its full antigenic reactivity. Most are due to discrete, genetically determined alterations in primary amino acid sequence, and other alterations in the physicochemical properties of the protein are likely to be present. If clinical abnormalities are present, they are indistinguishable from those observed when the protein is normal but present in markedly decreased amounts. Because the abnormal protein is antigenically reactive and its concentration in plasma is usually normal, its presence is not detected immunochemically, and a functional assay must be used. Because of this limitation, in a number of clinically important serum protein deficiencies, immunochemical measurements are not ideal for screening, although they are very helpful in defining the abnormality further, once a functional deficiency has been identified.

Despite the existing limitation, it is quite possible that more extensive studies will eventually provide antibodies that are more suitable for screening. Judging from the recent success in preparing antibodies that are specific for idiotypic determinants on gamma globulin molecules, in or near the specific combining sites of the antibody, it may also be possible to obtain antibodies to the catalytically active regions of normal clotting and complement proteins. By using such antibodies, the likelihood that a functionally inactive protein would retain its full immunological reactivity would be considerably reduced.

SUMMARY

1. Immunoassays suffer from many of the problems in interpretation that arise when any quantitative assay is used to estimate the pharmacologic or physiological response in the organism as a whole.

2. Immunoassay measurements are convenient for large-scale screening, particularly if measurements are made of overall antigenic reactivity and unfractionated tissue extracts are used. However, this practice is

predicated on the assumption that immunologically cross-reacting mole-cules are either absent or are present in quantities too small to interfere significantly in the immunoassay. However, in the unlikely event that unexpectedly high concentrations of cross-reactivity were present, the immunoassay results might well be misleading.

3. In congenital plasma protein deficiency states, a functionally in-active protein may retain its full antigenic reactivity, thus decreasing the value of immunological measurements for initial screening.

Chapter 13

Concluding Remarks. Present and Future Applications of Immunoassays

---

Since the early 1960s radioimmunoassays and other competitive binding assays have been developed to a remarkable array of biochemically or pharmacologically important substances and in many instances have virtually replaced other methods of measurement. It seems highly probable that this rapid rate of progress will continue, for numerous substances presently measured by other methods might, in principle, be measured with increased sensitivity and convenience by competitive binding techniques. This chapter will survey important existing applications of competitive binding measurements and attempt to project what some of the important future developments might be.

ENDOCRINOLOGY

The applications of competitive binding assays to the field of endocrinology have been reviewed extensively in Margoulies (1969) and Odell and Daughaday (1971). Among the early applications in this field were immunoassays for insulin (Yalow and Berson, 1960), T4 (Ekins, 1960), glucagon (Unger, Eisentraut, McCall, and Madison, 1961), growth hormone (Utiger, Parker, and Daughaday, 1962; Glick, Yalow, Berson, and Roth, 1963) TSH (Utiger, Odell, and Condliffe, 1963), PTH (Berson, Yalow, Aurbach, and Potts, 1963), corticosteroids (Murphy, Engelberg, and Patee, 1963), HCG (Paul and Odell, 1964; Midgley and Ram, 1965); ACTH, Yalow, Glick, Roth, and Berson, 1964), bradykinin (Goodfriend, Levine, and Fasman, 1964), angiotensin II (Goodfriend, Levine, and Fasman, 1964; Haber, Page, and Jacoby, 1965), prolactin (Beck, Parker, and Daughaday, 1965; Grumbach and Kaplan, 1964) and vasopressin (Permutt, Parker, and Utiger, 1966; Roth, Glick, Klein, and Peterson, 1966). In subsequent years radioimmunoassays have been developed for all the other major hormones, including α-MSH, β-MSH, LH,

FSH, human chorionic mammotropin, T_3, mineralocorticoids, estrogens, progesterones, androgens, oxytocin, calcitonin, gastrin, secretin, cholescystokinin-pancreozymin, cAMP, cGMP, prostaglandins, thyrotropin-releasing hormone, and LH-releasing hormone. In many instances, assays have been developed to the same hormone in different species or to different molecular forms of the hormone, so the total number of assay systems on which productive work has been done is actually considerably larger.

Some of the important general applications of immunoassays to endocrinologic studies are as follows:

1. In providing quantitative clinical laboratory measurements for the differential diagnosis of endocrine disorders.

2. In the performance of studies on the physiological and pharmacological control of hormone secretion and degradation.

3. In analyzing different hormones for areas of partial structural homology.

4. In determining the hormonal content of different tissues.

5. In determining whether the same hormones can circulate in different molecular forms.

6. In studies of the effect of antihormone antibodies on hormone activity and metabolism.

7. In the recognition and investigation of endocrine-secreting tumors.

8. In localizing endocrine-secreting glands or tumors in vivo in preparation for surgery.

The present widespread use of hormone immunoassays will undoubtedly continue. Although all the major hormones have presumably been elucidated and immunoassays already developed, additional hormones with a regional site of action analogous to the recently discovered hormones involved in communication between the hypothalamus and the pituitary may yet be uncovered, particularly in the central nervous system. One important future research direction is likely to be an increasing emphasis on selective immunochemical absorption techniques for purifying and concentrating hormones so that highly diluted samples can be measured. Such techniques would provide important new information regarding the physiological control and function of hormones presently measured only with considerable difficulty under normal physiological conditions (e.g., the vasopressins and bradykinin). It is probable that much attention will also be placed on the development of tissue-receptor-binding assays, but whether major advantages will accrue over existing hormone immunoassays remains to be seen.

PHARMACOLOGY

Applications of competitive binding measurements to pharmacology have been reviewed in detail by Marks, Morris, and Teale (1974). Among the early contributions in this field were immunoassays for digitoxin (Oliver, Parker, Brasfield, and Parker, 1966, 1968), cAMP and cGMP (Steiner, Kipnis, Utiger, and Parker, 1969), and morphine (Spector and Parker, 1970). Immunoassays have subsequently been applied to the measurement of other cardiac glycosides, prostaglandins, barbiturates, dilantin, gentamycin, LSD, chlorpromazine, tubocurarine, folic acid, vitamin A, vitamin D, amphetamines, normetanephrine, and pentazocine.

Some of the important general applications of immunological measurements to pharmacology include the following:

1. In providing rapid and convenient screening procedures for detection of drug abuse.

2. In the diagnosis of suspected drug poisoning.

3. In monitoring routine drug therapy with drugs subject to uncertain absorption or metabolism.

4. In the investigation of drug absorption, distribution, metabolism, and excretion.

5. In studies on the effect of antidrug antibodies on drug activity and toxicity.

6. In following changes in intracellular metabolism in response to drugs.

The development of new immunoassays for drugs could be rather a mixed blessing. On the one hand, a number of medically important drugs vary sufficiently in their absorption, metabolism, and excretion to merit regular measurements by immunoassay or some other method. Radioimmunoassays should be very valuable in this situation, particularly if the drug is difficult to measure by other techniques. On the other hand, there is nothing to indicate that the majority of drugs need to be monitored during therapy, and the possible cost of widespread and possibly unnecessary measurements must be kept in mind. Just how practical immunoassays will be in the routine monitoring of blood levels will depend in part on whether drug immunoassays can be further simplified and automated. The development of techniques that would permit rapid screening for the presence or absence of multiple drugs simultaneously, as would be desirable in suspected acute drug overdosage, also requires further attention. Immunochemical techniques are likely to see increasing application for forensic screening and in the rapid detection of hazardous contaminants in the environment.

INFECTIOUS DISEASES

Although immunological techniques have long been applied to the detection of antimicrobial antibodies, the application of sensitive immunological measurements to the detection of microbial antigens in vivo is of much more recent origin. The most important application has been the development of a sensitive radioimmunoassay for hepatitis B antigen (Walsh, Yalow, and Berson, 1970; Aach, Grisham, and Parker, 1971), which was subsequently applied to the subtyping of hepatitis B antigen (Aach, Hacker, and Parker, 1973; Ginsberg, Bancroft, and Conrad, 1972). Immunological techniques have also been used in rapid screening for bacterial antigens in suspected acute bacterial meningitis, although radioimmunoassays per se have not yet been used for this purpose.

From the limited data already available, it is apparent that

1. Radioimmunoassay screening methods can be used to monitor for microbial contamination in products intended for human use.

2. Sensitive immunological methods for microbial antigens can sometimes provide a rapid etiologic diagnosis in suspected acute infection, · thereby avoiding the delay required to obtain a definitive increase in antibody titer or to culture the microorganism.

3. Because of their ability to detect relatively minor antigen subtypes, radioimmunoassays provide a particularly powerful approach to studies of the epidemiology of human infections.

4. Radioimmunoassays can also be used to quantitate antibacterial agents, as discussed in the pharmacology section.

As for the future, certainly the use of highly sensitive immunological methods to detect microbial infections will be rapidly extended. It seems likely that radioimmunoassays will be applied on a very broad scale to the diagnosis of acute or chronic infections, both in screening for microbial antigens in blood, tissue, or urine and as a more sensitive and convenient means of detecting antibodies to microorganisms or their products. In particular, it seems very possible that chronic bacterial, viral, and parasitic diseases currently detected in part by delayed hypersensitivity testing or relatively insensitive serologic methods might be better diagnosed by radioimmunoassay. Attempts to demonstrate microbial or parasitic antigens in concentrates of serum, urine, or serous fluid would be of particular interest, since the quantity of antigen released by an infectious agent might be expected to correlate better with the existence of active infection than the degree of cellular or humoral immunity. Whether the levels of antigen released will be sufficient to permit this kind of analysis in all the infections of interest remains to be established. Even though circulating antigen is detected in almost all individuals having an acute hepatitis B virus infection and in whom blood is obtained at the appropriate time, since viremia is a hallmark of the disease, this may be an unusually favorable situation for detecting circulating antigen. Part of the problem will be the antigenic complexity of many of these agents, making it difficult to decide what the most important antigens to measure are; this subject will require further study.

In addition to measurements of microbial antigens and antimicrobial antibodies, assays for bacterial products may be useful. Evidence already exists that antibody formation is possible to endotoxin (Kataoka, Inoue, Galanos, and Kinsky, 1971; and if a sensitive immunoassay for endotoxin can be developed, it should have applicability in the diagnosis of acute endotoxin shock. Finally, recent preliminary studies with human leukocytic pyrogen (Wolfe and Parker, unpublished observations) suggest that it may be possible to raise antibodies to leukocytic pyrogen, which would create exciting new possibilities in the clinical diagnosis of fever.

CLINICAL IMMUNOLOGY

Radioimmunoassays have found a variety of applications in clinical immunology. Among the early contributions were immunoassays for individual immunoglobulin classes and subclasses (Fahey, 1963), for IgG anti-penicilloyl antibodies (Thiel, Mitchell, and Parker, 1964), for IgE antibodies to inhalant allergens (Wide, Bennich, and Johansson, 1967) and for anti-DNA antibodies (Wold, Young, Tan, and Farr, 1968). Further applications have included measurements of thyroglobulin antibodies, amyloidlike proteins, rheumatoid factors, complement components, and antibodies to food antigens.

As for the future, important new applications can be anticipated in the use of immunoassays for transplantation antigen typing, where the virtual lack of completely specific antibodies and the complex mosaic of antigens that must be screened have created serious problems in analysis. There is good reason to believe that radioimmunoassays would be highly useful in this setting, since they are susceptible to precise quantitation, require only very small amounts of antigen and antibody, and provide highly useful information about cross-reactivity. Although the preparation of soluble transplantation antigens for radiolabeling may present problems, already several reports indicate that radioimmunoassays have potential for histo-compatibility antigen typing (e.g., Foschi and Manson, 1970). More wide-spread use of radioimmunoassays for the diagnosis of allergy also seems likely, although at present the large number of antigens that must be screened in a routine allergic workup is a problem and will remain so until there is further progress toward automation. The development of reliable in vitro assays for drug allergy would be of particular value, since there has been a long delay in getting skin-test antigens of known effectiveness in penicillin allergy authorized for testing in vivo in human beings, and this same situation could arise in other drug allergies. Increasing activity can be anticipated in the complement field, as exemplified by the develop-ment of a radioimmunoassay for properdin (Minta et al., 1973).

One of the most interesting applications of immunoassays may be in the measurement and definition of various factors emanating from stim-ulated lymphocytes, mast cells, basophiles, phagocytic cells, platelets, and serum proteins when immunologc inflammation is initiated. In a sense, immunology may be at the same stage of development that endocrinology was 15 years ago in that there are a variety of factors, most of them poorly characterized, which are released at various stages of immune inflammation and which are capable of transmitting information to other cells. Although some are already characterized, enough work has already been done with the others to make it probable that further progress will be difficult. If sensitive radioimmunoassays could be developed, they would provide a valuable research tool for future studies.

HEMATOLOGY AND ONCOLOGY

Applications of competitive binding assays in hematology and oncology have been reviewed by Newmark and Gordon (1974) and Bagshawe (1974). Among the early applications in this field were assays for vitamin B_{12} (Rothenberg, 1961; Barakat and Ekins, 1961), carcinoembryonic antigen (Thomson et al., 1969), plasminogen (Rabiner, Goldfine, Hart, Summaria and Robbins, 1968), and fibrinogen and fibrin degradation products (Catt, Hirsh, Castelan, Niall, and Tregear, 1968). Additional applications include measurements of erythropoietin, blood group antigens, antibodies to platelets, red cells and clotting factors, clotting and comple-ment proteins, ferritin, transferrin, plasmin, folic acid, intrinsic factor, transcobalbumin, and α-fetoprotein.

As discussed in Chapter 12, important new areas of immunoassay de-velopment in hematology will be in the quantitative measurement of com-plement and clotting factors, particularly if antibodies can be obtained that measure activated proteins in the presence of large quantities of their protein precursors. Partial success in this regard has already been achieved by Rabiner and his colleagues (1969) with plasminogen and plasmin. The availability of antibodies with more refined specificities might also make it feasible to use antibodies to screen for quantitatively normal but functionally inactive circulating proteins (see Chapter 12).

In the tumor immunology area, the further extension of immunoassay applications seems strongly indicated on the basis of the established usefulness of radioimmunoassay meaurements of HCG, carcinoembryonic antigen, and α-fetoprotein in the initial screening and postoperative followup of tumors that release these proteins. Although none of these proteins is absolutely specific for malignancy, nonetheless, they provide useful information, particularly in the diagnosis of tumor recurrence. Just how useful immunoassay screening procedures will be for other tumors will depend primarily on how successful further attempts at identification of human tumor associated or tumor specific antigens turn out to be.

CARDIOLOGY

Although immunoassay applications to cardiology have largely centered on the detection of digitalis toxicity up to now, an important new application can be foreseen in the monitoring of blood levels of antiarrhythmic drugs. Another potential application would be in the measurement of enzymes released into the plasma during myocardial damage, such as creatine phosphokinase (CPK). CPK has a sufficiently specific isozymal pattern in the heart that the pattern of circulating CPK isozymes would be expected to change during myocardial necrosis.

ORGAN PHYSIOLOGY

Immunological detection methods have an important future in evaluating structure-function relationships in highly complex organs, such as the brain (or as noted above, responding lymphocyte tissues), where the cells are heterogenous and a variety of mechanisms of intercellular communication may exist.

MOLECULAR BIOLOGY

The ability of antibodies to determine where antigens are localized in cells is well recognized, based on the immunofluorescence studies of Coons and others, and has given rise to important new concepts of how cells function biochemically, as, for example, the recent demonstration by immunofluorescence using anti-cAMP antibodies that cAMP appears to be generated in different parts of the lymphocyte in response to different adenylate cyclase-stimulating agents (Bloom, Wedner, and Parker, 1973). The use of antibodies to purify, measure, and characterize subcellular fractions of cells is only beginning to be exploited. For instance, among the new immunological reagents currently being developed are antibodies capable of localizing and quantitating microfilaments and microtubular elements inside cells. Antibodies are also beginning to be used to probe the structure of chromatin and other nuclear elements and to detect intracellular virus or virus specified proteins. These are only a few of the new applications of immunochemical techniques that can be foreseen in the molecular biology area.

References

Aach, R. D., J. W. Grisham, and C. W. Parker. 1971. Proc. Nat. Acad. Sci. USA. 68:1056.

Aach, R. D., E. J. Hacker, and C. W. Parker. 1973. J. Immun., 111:381.

Abraham, G. E., and P. K. Grover. 1971. *In* W. D. Odell, and W. H. Daughaday (Eds.). Principles of competitive protein-binding assays. J. B. Lippincott Co., Philadelphia. p. 134.

Ada, G. L., C. R. Parrish, G. J. V. Nossal, and A. Abbot. 1967. Cold Spring Harbor Symposia on Quantitative Biology. 32:381.

Adler, F. L., C. Liu, and D. H. Catlin. 1972. Clinical Immunology and Immunopathology. 1:53.

Alexander, N. M. 1974. J. Biol. Chem. 249:1946.

Anderer, F. A., and H. D. Schlumberger. 1965. Biochim. Biophys. Acta. 97:503.

Arnon, R., and M. Sela. 1969. Proc. Nat. Acad. Sci. USA. 62:163.

Arquilla, E. K., and J. Finn. 1965. J. Exp. Med. 122:771.

Atassi, M. Z., and B. J. Saplin, 1968, Biochemistry. 7:688.

Bagshawe, K. D. 1974. Brit. Med. Bull. 30:68.

Barakat, R. M., and R. P. Ekins. 1961. Lancet. 2:25.

Barrett, J. T. 1965. Immunology. 8:128.

Beck, P., M. L. Parker, and W. H. Daughaday. 1965. J. Clin. Endocr. 25:1457.

Benjamini, E., M. Shimizu, J. D. Young, and C. Y. Leung. 1968. Biochemistry. 7:1253.

Benjamini, E., J. D. Young, W. J. Peterson, C. Y. Leung, and M. Shimizu. 1965. Biochemistry. 4:2081.

Berson, S. A., and R. S. Yalow. 1958. Advances Biol. Med. Phys. 6:349.

Berson, S. A., R. S. Yalow, G. D. Aurbach, and J. T. Potts. 1963. Proc. Nat. Acad. Sci. USA. 49:613.

215

Berson, S. A., R. S. Yalow, M. A. Bauman, M. A. Rothschild, and K. Newerly. 1956. J. Clin. Invest. 35:170.

Berson, S. A., R. S. Yalow, S. S. Schreiber, and J. Post. 1953. J. Clin. Invest. 32:746.

Bloom, F. E., H. J. Wedner, and C. W. Parker. 1973. Pharmacol. Rev. 25:343.

Boden, G. 1974. In B. M. Jaffe and H. R. Behrman (Eds.). Methods of hormone radioimmunoassay. Academic Press, New York. P. 275.

Bogdanove, E. M., N. B. Schwartz, L. E. Reichert, and A. R. Midgley. 1971. Endocrinology. 88:644.

Bolton, A. E., and W. M. Hunter. 1973. Biochem. J. 133:529.

Boyd, G. W., and W. S. Peart. 1968. Lancet. 2:129.

Brenneman, L., and S. J. Singer. 1968. Proc. Nat. Acad. Sci. USA. 60:258.

Brown, R. K. 1962. J. Biol. Chem. 237:1162.

Brown, R. F., R. Delaney, L. Levine, and H. Van Vunakis. 1959. J. Biol. Chem. 234:2043.

Brumbaugh, P. F., D. H. Haussler, R. Bressler, and M. R. Haussler. 1974. Science. 183:1089.

Burr, I. M., P. C. Sizonenko, S. L. Kaplan, and M. M. Gruinback. 1969. J. Clin. Endocr. 29:691.

Butler, V. P., S. M. Beiser, B. F. Erlanger, S. W. Tanenbaum, S. Cohen, and A. Bendich. 1962. Proc. Nat. Acad. Sci. USA. 48:1597.

Butt, W. R. 1972. J. Endocr. 55:453.

Cailla, H. L., M. S. Racine-Weisbuch, and M. A. Delaage. 1973. Anal. Biochem. 56:394.

Catch, J. R. 1971. In Y. Cohen (Ed.). International encyclopedia of pharmacology and therapeutics. Pergammon Press, Oxford. p. 97.

Catt, K. J., 1970, Acta Endocr. Second Supp. 142:222.

Catt, K. J., J. Hirsh, D. J. Castelan, H. D. Niall, and G. W. Tregear. 1968. Thromb. Diath. Haemorrh. 20:1.

Cebra, J. J. 1961. J. Immunol. 86:205.

Ceska, M., A. V. Sjodin, and F. Grossmüller. 1971. Biochem. J. 121:139.

Challand, G., D. Goldie, and J. Landon. 1974. Brit. Med. Bull. 30:18.

Copeland, E. S. 1973. Ann. N.Y. Acad. Sci. 222:1097.

Cotes, P. M., M. V. Mussett, and I. Berryman. 1969. J. Endocr. 45:557.

Crumpton, M. J., and J. M. Wilkinson. 1965. Biochem. J. 94:545.

Cuatrecasas, P. 1971. Proc. Nat. Acad. Sci. USA. 68:1264.

Cvoric, J. 1969. J. Chromatogr. 44:349

Dandliker, W. B., and V. A. de Saussure. 1970. Immunochemistry. 7:799.

David, G. S. 1972. Biochem. Biophys. Res. Commun. 48:464.

David, J. R., and S. F. Schlossman. 1968. J. Exp. Med. 128:1451.

Day, L. A., J. M. Sturtevant, and S. J. Singer. 1963. Ann. N.Y. Acad. Sci. 103:611.

Dresser, D. W. 1962. Immunology. 5:161.

Egan, M. L., J. T. Lautenschleger, J. E. Coligan, and C. W. Todd. 1972. Immunochemistry. 9:289.

Eisen, H. N. 1959. In H. S. Lawrence (Ed.). Cellular and humoral aspects of the hypersensitive states, P. B. Hoeber, Inc., New York. p. 89.

Eisen, H. N. 1966. Harvey lectures. 60:1.

Eisen, H. N., and F. Karush. 1949. J. Amer. Chem. Soc. 71:363.

Eisen, H. N., and G. W. Siskind. 1964. Biochemistry. 3:996.

Eisen, H. N., E. S. Simms, J. R. Little, and L. A. Steiner. 1964 Fed. Proc. 23:559.

Eisen, S. A., L. R. Lyle, and C. W. Parker. 1971. Fed. Proc. 30:649.

Ekins, R. P. 1960. Clin. Chim. Acta. 5:453.

Ekins, R. P. 1974. Brit. Med. Bull. 30:3.

Ekins, R. P., G. B. Newman, and J. L. H. O'Riordan. 1968. In R. L. Hayes, F. A. Goswitz, and B. E. P. Murphy (Eds.). Radioisotopes in medicine: In vitro studies, U.S. Atomic Energy Commission, Oak Ridge. p. 59.

Ekins, R. P., G. B. Newman, and J. L. H. O'Riordan. 1970. In J. W. McArther, and T. Colton (Eds.). Statistics in endocrinology, MIT Press, Cambridge. p. 345.

Erlanger, B. F. 1973. Pharmacol. Rev. 25:271.

Evans, E. A. 1966. Nature. 209:169.

Fahey, J. L. 1963. J. Immunol. 91:438.

Farr, R. S. 1958. J. Infect. Dis. 103:239.

Farr, R. S. 1971. In C. A. Williams, and M. W. Chase (Eds.). Methods in immunology and immunochemistry. Vol. III. Academic Press, New York. p. 66.

Feldman, H., and D. Rodbard. 1971. *In* W. D. Odell, and W. H. Daughaday (Eds.). Principles of competitive protein-binding assays. J. B. Lippincott Co., Philadelphia. p. 158.

Fischer, J. A., U. Binswanger, and F. M. Dietrich. 1974. J. Clin. Invest. 54:1382.

Foschi, G. V., and L. A. Manson. 1970. Nautre. 225:853.

Freedlender, A. E. 1969. *In* M. Margoulies (Ed.). Protein and polypeptide hormones, Excerpta Med. Fdn, Amsterdam. pp. 351-354, 611, 670-671.

Freedlender, A. E., and R. E. Cathou. 1971. *In* K. E. Kirkham, and W. M. Hunter (Eds.). Radioimmunoassay methods, Churchill Livingstone, Edinburgh. p. 94.

Freedman, M. H., and M. Sela. 1966. J. Biol. Chem. 241:2382.

Freedman, M. H., A. L. Grossberg, and D. Pressman. 1968. Biochemistry. 7:1941.

Frei, P. C., B. Benacerraf, and G. J. Thorbecke. 1965. Proc. Nat. Acad. Sci. USA. 53:20.

Frey, J. R., A. L. de Weck, H. T. Geleick, and W. Lergier. 1969. J. Exp. Med. 130:1123.

Froese, A. 1968. Immunochemistry. 5:253.

Froese, A., and A. H. Sehon. 1965. Immunochemistry. 2:135.

Fujio, H., and F. Karush. 1966. Biochemistry. 5:1856.

Gavin, J. R., P. Gorden, J. Roth, J. A. Archer, and D. N. Buell. 1973. J. Biol. Chem. 248:2202.

Gavin, J. R., J. Roth, P. Jen, and P. Freychet. 1972. Proc. Nat Acad. Sci. USA. 69:747.

Gill, G. N., and L. D. Garren. 1969. Proc. Nat. Acad. Sci. USA. 63:512.

Gill, T. J., H. W. Kunz, and P. S. Marfey. 1965. J. Biol. Chem. 240:3227.

Gilliland, P. F., and T. E. Prout. 1965. Metabolism. 14:918.

Gilman, A. G. 1970. Proc. Nat. Acad. Sci. USA. 67:305.

Ginsberg, A. L., W. H. Bancroft, and M. E. Conrad. 1972. J. Lab. Clin. Med. 80:291.

Glick, S. M., R. S. Yalow, S. A. Berson, and J. Roth. 1963. Nature. 199:784.

Goodfriend, T. L. 1975. Personal communication.

Goodfriend, T. L., and D. L. Ball. 1969. J. Lab. Clin. Med. 73:501.

Goodfriend, T. L., and C. E. Odya. 1974. *In* B. M. Jaffe, and H. R. Behrman (Eds.). Methods of hormone radioimmunoassay. Academic Press, New York. p. 439

Goodfriend, T., L. Levine, and G. D. Fasman. 1964. Science. 144:1344.

Goodman, J. W., D. E. Nitechi, and I. M. Stoltenberg. 1968. Biochemistry. 7:706.

Grant, G. H., and W. R. Butt. 1970. *In* O. Bodansky, and C. P. Stewart (Eds.). Advances in clinical chemistry. Vol. 13. Academic Press, New York. p. 430.

Greenwood, F. C. 1971. *In* W. D. Odell, and W. H. Daughaday (Eds.). Principles of competitive protein-binding assays. J. B. Lippincott Co., Philadelphia. p. 288.

Grey, N., J. E. McGuigan, and D. M. Kipnis. 1970. Endocrinol. 86:1383.

Grodsky, G. M., and P. H. Forsham. 1960. J. Clin. Invest. 39:1070.

Grumbach, M. M., and S. L. Kaplan. 1964-1965. Trans. N.Y. Acad. Sci. 27:167.

Haber, E. 1964. Proc. Nat. Acad. Sci. 52:1099.

Haber, E. 1969. N. Eng. J. Med. 280:148.

Haber, E., L. B. Page, and G. A. Jacoby. 1965. Biochemistry (Wash.). 4:693.

Haber, E., F. F. Richards, and L. B. Page. 1965. Anal. Biochem. 12:163.

Halloran, M. J., and C. W. Parker. 1964. J. Lab. Clin. Med. 64:865 (abstract).

Halloran, M. J., and C. W. Parker. 1966. J. Immunol. 96:373.

Harel, S., S. Ben-Efraim, and P. Liacopoulos. 1970. Immunology. 19:319.

Hendrick, J. C., J. J. Legros, and P. Franchimont. 1971. Ann. Endocr. 32:241.

Herbert, V. 1969. *In* M. Margoulies (Ed.). Protein and polypeptide hormones, Excerpta Medica Fdn., Amsterdam. p. 55.

Hichens, M., P. H. Gale, and H. Schwam. 1974. *In* B. M. Jaffe, and H. R. Behrman (Eds.). Methods of hormone radioimmunoassay. Academic Press, New York. 1974. p. 45.

Holohan, K. N., R. F. Murphy, R. W. J. Flanagan, K. D. Buchanan, and D. T. Elmore. 1973. Biochim. Biophys. Acta. 322:178.

Hornick, C. L., and F. Karush. 1969. *In* M. Sela, and M. Prywes (Eds.). Topics in basic immunology. Academic Press, New York. p. 29.

Hsia, J. C., and L. H. Piette. 1969. Arch. Biochem. Biophys. 132:466.

Hunter, W. M. 1967. *In* D. M. Weir, (Ed.). Handbook of experimental immunology. Blackwell Scientific Publications, Oxford. p. 608.

Hunter, W. M. 1973. *In* D. M. Weir (Ed.). Handbook of experimental immunology. 2nd ed. Blackwell Scientific Publications, Oxford. p. 17.1.

Hunter, W. M. 1974. Brit. Med. Bull. 30:18.

Hunter, W. H., and F. C. Greenwood. 1962. Nature. 194:495.

Hurwitz, E., S. Fuchs, and M. Sela. 1965. Biochim. Biophys. Acta. 111:512.

Isersky, C., H. Metzger, and D. Buell. 1975. J. Exp. Med. 141:1147.

Ishizaka, T., D. H. Campbell, and K. Ishizaka. 1960. Proc. Soc. Exp. Biol. Med. 103:5.

Jacobs, L. S., I. K. Mariz, and W. H. Daughaday. 1972. J. Clin. Endocr. 34:484.

Jaffe, B. M., and H. R. Behrman. 1974. *In* B. M. Jaffe, and H. R. Behrman (Eds.). Methods of hormone radioimmunoassay. Academic Press, New York. p. 19.

Jaffe, B. M., and J. H. Walsh. 1974. *In* B. M. Jaffe, and H. R. Behrman (Eds.). Methods of hormone radioimmunoassay. Academic Press, New York. p. 251.

Jaffe, B. M., H. R. Behrman, and C. W. Parker. 1973. J. Clin. Invest. 52:398.

Jaffe, B. M., W. T. Newton, and J. E. McGuigan. 1970. Immunochemistry. 7:715.

Jaffe, B. M., J. W. Smith, W. T. Newton, and C. W. Parker. 1971. Science. 171:494.

Jirousek, L., and E. T. Pritchard, 1971. Biochim. Biophys. Acta. 243:230.

Johnson, H. M., K. Brenner, and H. E. Hull. 1966. J. Immunol. 97:791.

Kabat E. A., 1954. J. Amer. Chem. Soc. 76:3709.

Karush, F., 1957. J. Amer. Chem. Soc. 79:3380.

Karush, F. 1962. *In* W. H. Taliaferro, and J. H. Humphrey (Eds.). Advances in immunology. Vol. 2. Academic Press, New York. p. 1.

Kataoka, T., K. Inoue, C. Galanos, and S. C. Kinsky. 1971. Eur. J. Biochem. 24:123.

Katchalski, E., M. Sela, H. I. Silman, and A. Berger. 1964. *In* H. Neurath (Ed.). The proteins. Vol. II, Academic Press, New York. p. 405.

Katz, D. H., and B. Benacerraf. 1972. *In* F. J. Dixon, and H. G. Kunkel (Eds.). Advances in immunology. Vol. 15. Academic Press, New York. p. 1.

Keck, K., A. L. Grossberg, and D. Pressman. 1973. Immunochemistry. 10:331.

Keston, A. S., and R. Brandt. 1965. Anal. Biochem. 11:1.

Kim, Y. T., N. Merrifield, T. Zarchy, N. I. Brody, and G. W. Siskind. 1974. Immunology. 26:943.

Kim, Y. T., and G. W. Siskind. 1974. Clin. Exp. Immunol. 17:329.

Kimball, J. W. 1972. Immunochemistry. 9:1169.

Kimura, H., and F. Murad. 1974. J. Biol. Chem. 249:329.

Knowles, J. R. 1972. Accounts of Chemical Research. 5:155.

Korenman, S. G. 1968. J. Clin. Endocr. 28:127.

Korenman, S. G., and B. A. Sanborn. 1971. In W. D. Odell, and W. H. Daughaday (Eds.). Principles of competitive protein-binding assays. J. B. Lippincott Co., Philadelphia. p. 89.

Koshland, M. E., and F. Englberger. 1963. Proc. Nat. Acad. Sci. USA. 50:61.

Koshland, M. E., J. J. Davis, and N. J. Fujita. 1969. Proc. Nat. Acad. Sci. USA. 63:1274.

Koshland, M. E., F. Englberger, and S. M. Gaddone. 1962. J. Immunol. 89:517.

Krause, R. M. 1970. Fed. Proc. 29:59.

Kreiter, V. P., and D. Pressman. 1964. Biochemistry. 3:274.

Lambert, B., and C. Jacquemin. 1973. Biochimie. 55:1395.

Landon, J., T. Livanou, and F. C. Greenwood. 1967. Biochem. J. 105:1075.

Landsteiner, K. 1936. Specificity of serological reactions. Charles C Thomas, Springfield, Ill.

Lee, C. Y., and R. J. Ryan. 1972. Proc. Nat. Acad. Sci. USA. 69:3520.

Lefkowitz, R. J., J. Roth, and I. Pastan. 1970. Science. 170:633.

Leray, F., A. Chambaut, M. Perrenoud, and J. Hanoune. 1973. Eur. J. Biochem. 38:185.

Leskowitz, S., V. E. Jones, and S. J. Zak. 1966. J. Exp. Med. 123:229.

Lesniak, M. A., P. Gorden, J. Roth, and J. R. Gavin. 1974. J. Biol. Chem. 249:1661.

Leute, R. 1973. Ann. N.Y. Acad. Sci. 222:1087.

Leute, R., E. F. Ullman, A. Goldstein, and L. A. Herzenberg. 1972. Nature New Biology. 236:93.

Levine, B. B. 1965. Fed. Proc. 24:45.

Levine, L., and H. Van Vunakis. 1970. Biochem. Biophys. Res. Commun. 41:1171.

Levine, L., R. M. Gutierrez-Cernosek, and H. Van Vunakis. 1971. J. Biol. Chem. 246:6782.

Little, J. R., and R. B. Counts. 1969. Biochemistry. 8:2729.

Little, J. R., and H. N. Eisen. 1966. Biochemistry. 5:3385.

Little, J. R., and H. N. Eisen. 1967. Biochemistry. 6:3119.

Lowry, O. H., and J. V. Passonneau. 1972. A flexible system of enzymatic analysis. Academic Press, New York.

Mamet-Bradley, M. D. 1966. Immunochemistry. 3:155.

Marcario, A. J. L., E. C. Marcario, C. Franceschi, and F. Celada. 1972. J. Exp. Med. 136:353.

Marchalonis, J. J. 1969. Biochem. J. 113:299.

Margoulies, M. (Ed.). 1969. Protein and polypeptide hormones. Excerpta Med. Fdn., Amsterdam.

Marks, V., B. A. Morris, and J. D. Teale. 1974. Brit. Med. Bull. 30:80.

Massaglia, U., R. Rialdi, and C. A. Rossi. 1969. Biochem. J. 115:11.

Matsukura, S., C. D. West, Y. Ichikawa, W. Jubiz, G. Harada, and F. H. Tyler. 1971. J. Lab. Clin. Med. 77:490.

Mayberry, W. E., J. E. Rall, M. Bernan, and D. Bertoli. 1965. Biochem. 4:1965.

Mayer, S. E., J. T. Stull, and W. B. Wastila. 1974. In J. G. Hardman, and B. W. O'Malley (Eds.). Methods in enzymology. Vol. 38. Part C. Academic Press, New York. p. 3.

McDevitt, H. O., and B. Benacerraf. 1969. Advances in Immunology. 11:31.

McFarlane, A. S. 1965. In Radioisotope techniques in the study of protein metabolism. International Atomic Energy Agency, Vienna. pp. 3-6.

Metzger, H. 1967. Proc. Nat. Acad. Sci. USA. 57:1490.

Midgley, A. R. 1969. In M. Margoulies (Ed.). Protein and Polypeptide hormones. Excerpta Medica Foundation, Amsterdam. p. 713.

Midgley, A. R., and J. S. Ram. 1965. Fed. Proc. Fed. Amer. Soc. Exp. Biol. 24:162.

Midgley, A. R., G. D. Niswender, V. L. Gay, and L. E. Reichert. 1971. Recent Progr. Hormones Res. 27:235.

Miles, L. E. M., and C. N. Hales. 1968. Biochem. J. 108:611.

Minta, J. O., I. Goodkofsky, and I. H. Lepow. 1973. Immunochemistry. 10:341.

Mitchison, N. A. 1967. Cold Spring Harbor Symposia on Quantitative Biology. 32:431.

Miyachi, Y., and A. Chrambach. 1972. Biochem. Biophys. Res. Commun. 46:1213.

Morrison, M., and G. S. Bayse. 1970. Biochemistry. 9:2995.

Morrison, M., and G. S. Bayse. 1974. In T. E. King, H. S. Mason, and M. Morrison (Eds.). Oxidases and related redox systems. Vol. I. University Park Press, Baltimore. p. 375.

Morrison, M., G. S. Bayse, and R. G. Webster. 1971. Immunochem. 8:289.

Murphy, B. E. P. 1971. In W. D. Odell, and W. H. Daughaday (Eds.). Principles of competitive protein-binding assays. J. B. Lippincott Co. Philadelphia. p. 108.

Murphy, B. E. P., W. Engelberg, and C. F. Pattee. 1963. J. Clin. Endocr. 23:293.

Newmark, P. A., and Y. B. Gordon. 1974. Brit. Med. Bull. 30:86.

Newton, W. T., J. E. McGuigan, and B. M. Jaffe. 1970. J. Lab. Clin. Med. 78:886.

Niederer, W. 1974. J. Immunol. Methods. 5:77.

Nisonoff, A., and D. Pressman. 1958. J. Immunol. 81:126.

Nisonoff, A., M. Reichlin, and E. Margoliash. 1970. J. Biol. Chem. 245:940.

Obermayer, F., and E. P. Pick. 1904. Wien, Klin. Wschr. 17:265.

Odell, W. D., and W. H. Daughaday (Eds.). 1971. Principles of competitive protein-binding assays. J. B. Lippincott Co., Philadelphia.

Odell, W. D., G. A. Abraham, W. R. Skowsky, M. A. Hescox, and D. A. Fisher. 1971. In W. D. Odell, and W. H. Daughaday (Eds.). Principles of competitive protein-binding assays. J. B. Lippincott Co., Philadelphia. p. 57.

Odell, W. D., J. F. Wilber, and R. D. Utiger. 1967. Recent Progr. Hormone Res. 23:47.

Oliver, G. C., D. Brasfield, B. M. Parker, and C. W. Parker. 1966 J. Lab. Clin. Med. 68:1002.

Oliver, G. C., B. M. Parker, and C. W. Parker. 1971. Amer. J. Med. 51:186.

Oliver, G. C., B. M. Parker, D. L. Brasfield, and C. W. Parker. 1968. J. Clin. Invest. 47:1035.

Orth, D. N. 1974. *In* B. M. Jaffe, and H. R. Behrman (Eds.). Methods of hormone radioimmunoassay. Academic Press, New York. p. 125.

Osler, A. G. 1971. *In* C. A. Williams, and M. W. Chase (Eds.). Methods in immunology and immunochemistry. Vol. III. Academic Press, New York. p. 73.

Parish, C. R., and P. Stanley. 1972. Immunochemistry. 9:853.

Parker, C. W. 1965*a*. Fed. Proc. 24:51.

Parker, C. W. 1965*b*. *In* H. L. Alexander, and M. Samter (Eds.). Immunological diseases. Little, Brown and Co., Boston. p. 663.

Parker, C. W. 1967. *In* D. M. Weir (Ed.). Handbook of experimental immunology. Blackwell Scientific Publications, Oxford. p. 423.

Parker, C. W. 1971. *In* W. D. Odell, and W. H. Daughaday (Eds.). Principles of competitive protein-binding assays. J. B. Lippincott Co., Philadelphia. p. 25.

Parker, C. W. 1972*a*. *In* L. Goldberg (Ed.). Critical reviews in toxicology. Vol. I. Issue 3. CRC Press, Cleveland. p. 261.

Parker, C. W. 1972*b*. *In* M. Stefanini (Ed.). Progress in clinical pathology. Vol. 4. Grune and Stratton, New York. p. 103.

Parker, C. W. 1973. *In* D. M. Weir (Ed.). Handbook of experimental immunology. Blackwell Scientific Publications, Oxford. p. 14.1.

Parker, C. W. 1974. *In* The poisoned patient: the role of the laboratory. Ciba Foundation Symposium 26. Associated Scientific Publishers, Amsterdam. p. 201.

Parker, C. W., and C. K. Osterland. 1970. Biochemistry. 9:1074.

Parker, C. W., S. M. Godt, and M. C. Johnson. 1966. Biochemistry. 5:2314.

Parker, C. W., S. M. Godt, and M. C. Johnson, 1967*a*. Biochemistry. 6:3417.

Parker, C. W., M. Kern, and H. N. Eisen. 1962. J. Exp. Med. 115:789.

Parker, C. W., J. A. Thiel, and S. Mitchell. 1965. J. Immunol. 94:289.

Parker, C. W., T. J. Yoo, M. C. Johnson, and S. M. Godt. 1967*b*. Biochemistry. 6:3408.

Parker, M. L., and W. H. Daughaday. 1964. J. Clin. Endocr. 24:997.

Paul, W. E., and W. D. Odell. 1964. Nature (London) 203:979.

Peake, G. T. 1974. *In* B. M. Jaffe and H. R. Behrman (Eds.). Methods of hormone radioimmunoassay. Academic Press, New York. p. 103.

Permutt, M. A., C. W. Parker, and R. D. Utiger. 1966. Endocrinology. 78:809.

Pierce, J. V., and M. E. Webster. 1966. *In* E. G. Erdös, N. Back., and F. Secutin (Eds.). Hypotensive peptides. Springer-Verlag, Berlin. p. 130.

Playfair, J. H. L., B. A. L. Hurn, and D. Schulster. 1974. Brit. Med. Bull. 30:24.

Plescia, O. J., W. Braun, and N. C. Palczuk. 1964. Proc. Nat. Acad. Sci. USA. 52:279.

Plow, E. F., and T. S. Edgington. 1973. Proc. Nat. Acad. Sci. USA. 70:1169.

Porter, R. R. 1957. Biochem. J. 66:677.

Prescott, L. F. 1974. *In* The poisoned patent: the role of the laboratory. Ciba Foundation Symposium 26. Associated Scientific Publishers, Amsterdam. (Remarks in discussion.) pp. 230-238.

Pressman, D., and H. N. Eisen. 1950. J. Immunol. 64:273.

Pressman, D., and A. L. Grossberg, 1968. The structural basis of antibody specificity. W. A. Benjamin, Inc., New York.

Rabiner, S. F., I. D. Goldfine, A. Hart, L. Summaria, and K. C. Robbins. 1969. J. Lab. Clin. Med. 74:265

Rajewsky, K., V. Schirrmacher, S. Nase, and N. K. Jerne. 1969. J. Exp. Med. 129:1131.

Ramachandran, L. K. 1956. Chemical Reviews. 56:199.

Rao, C. V. 1974. J. Biol. Chem. 249:2864.

Ratcliffe, J. G. 1974. Brit. Med. Bull. 30:32.

Rehfeld, J. F., and F. Stadil. 1973. Scand. J. Clin. Lab. Invest. 31:459.

Reiss, E., and J. M. Canterbury. 1969. New Eng. J. Med. 280:1381.

Repke, D. W., and J. E. Zull. 1972. J. Biol. Chem. 247:2189.

Ricketts, C. R. 1966. Nature. 210:1113.

Riesen, W. and V. Castel. 1973. Experientia. 29:608.

Rodbard, D. 1971. *In* W. D. Odell, and W. H. Daughaday (Eds.). Principles of competitive protein-binding assays. J. B. Lippincott Co., Philadelphia. p. 204.

Rodbard, D., and G. H. Weiss. 1973. Anal. Biochem. 52:10.

Rodbard, D., P. L. Rayford, J. A. Cooper, and J. T. Ross. 1968. J. Clin. Endocr. 28:1412.

Rodbell, M., L. Birnbaumer, S. L. Pohl, and H. M. J. Krans. 1971. J. Biol. Chem. 246:1877.

Root, M. A., R. E. Chance, and J. A. Galloway. 1972. Diabetes. 21 (Suppl. 2):657.

Rosa, U., F. Pennisi, R. Bianchi, and K. Donato. 1967. Biochim. Biophys. Acta. 133:486.

Roth, J., S. M. Glick, L. A. Klein, and M. J. Petersen. 1966. J. Clin. Endocr. 26:671.

Rothenberg, S. P. 1961. Proc. Soc. Exp. Biol. Med. 108:45.

Rubenstein, K. E., R. S. Schneider, and E. F. Ullman. 1972. Biochem. Biophys. Res. Commun. 47:846.

Ryan, R. J., 1969. Acta Endocrinol. (Copenhagen) suppl. no. 142, p. 300.

Sage, H. J., G. F. Deutsch, G. D. Fasman, and L. Levine. 1964. Immuno-chemistry 1:133.

Scherberg, N. H., and S. Refetoff. 1974. J. Biol. Chem. 249:2143.

Schmidt, D. H., B. M. Kaufman, and V. P. Butler. 1974. J. Exp. Med. 139:278.

Segre, D., and M. Segre. 1973. Science. 181:851.

Sela, M., and E. Mozes. 1966. Proc. Nat. Acad. Sci. USA. 55:445.

Sela, M., B. Schechter, I. Schechter, and F. Borek. 1967. Cold Spring Harbor Symposia on Quantitative Biology. 32:537.

Sherman, L. A., S. Harwig, and O. A. Hayne. 1974. Int. J. Appl. Radiat. 25:81.

Singer, S. J. 1964. Immunochemistry. 1:15.

Siskind, G. W., W. E. Paul, and B. Benaceraf. 1967. Immunochemistry. 4:455.

Smith, T. W., V. P. Butler, and E. Haber. 1969. New Eng. J. Med. 281:1212.

Sobey, W. R., and K. M. Adams. 1961. Aust. J. Biol. Sci. 14:588.

Spector, S., and C. W. Parker. 1970. Science. 168:1347.

Spector, S., B. Berkowitz, E. J. Flynn, and B. Peskar. 1973. Pharmacol. Rev. 25:281.

Steiner, A. L. 1974. In B. M. Jaffe, and H. R. Behrman (Eds.). Methods of hormone radioimmunoassay. Academic Press, New York. p. 3.

Steiner, A. L., D. M. Kipnis, R. Utiger, and C. W. Parker. 1969. Proc. Nat. Acad. Sci. USA. 64:367.

Steiner, A. L., C. W. Parker, and D. M. Kipnis. 1970. In P. Greengard, and E. Costa (Eds.). Advances in biochemical psychopharmacology. Vol. III. Raven Press, New York. p. 89.

Steiner, A. L., C. W. Parker, and D. M. Kipnis. 1972. J. Biol. Chem. 247:1106.

Steiner, D. F., S. Cho, C. Bayliss, and O. Hallund. 1968. Diabetes. 17 (Suppl. 1):309.

Steiner, L. A., and H. N. Eisen. 1967. J. Exp. Med. 126:1161.

Stryer, L., and O. H. Griffith. 1965. Proc. Nat. Acad. Sci. USA. 54:1785.

Sunshine, I. 1974. *In* The poisoned patient: the role of the laboratory. Ciba Foundation Symposium 26. Associated Scientific Publishers, Amsterdam. p. 193.

Talamo, R. C., E. Haber, and K. F. Austen. 1969. J. Lab. Clin. Med. 74:816.

Thiel, J. A., S. Mitchell, and C. W. Parker. 1964. J. Allergy. 35:399.

Thompson, K. E., and J. G. Levy. 1970. Biochemistry. 9:3463.

Thomson, D. M. P., U. Krupey, S. O. Freedman, and P. Gold. 1969. Proc. Nat. Acad. Sci. USA. 64:161.

Thorell, J. I., and B. Johansson. 1971. Biochem. Biophys. Acta. 251:363.

Tigelaar, R. E., R. L. Rapport, J. K. Inman, and H. J. Kupferberg. 1973. Clin. Chim. Acta. 43:231.

Timpl, R., H. Furthmayr, and W. Beil. 1972. J. Immunol. 108:119.

Underdown, B. J., and H. N. Eisen. 1971. J. Immunol. 106:1431.

Unger, R. H., A. M. Eisentraut, M. S. McCall, and L. L. Madison. 1961. J. Clin. Invest. 40:1280.

Unger, R. H., A. M. Eisentraut, M. S. McCall, S. Keller, H. C. Lanz, and L. L. Madison. 1959. Proc. Soc. Exp. Biol. Med. 102:621.

Urbain, J., A. Van Acker, C. De Vos-Cloetens, and G. U. Urbain-Vansanten. 1972. Immunochemistry. 9:121.

Utiger, R. D. 1974. *In* B. M. Jaffe, and H. R. Behrman (Eds.). Methods of hormone radioimmunoassay. Academic Press, New York. p. 161.

Utiger, R. D., W. D. Odell, and P. G. Condlifle. 1963. Endocrinology. 73:359.

Utiger, R. D., M. L. Parker, and W. H. Daughaday. 1962. J. Clin. Invest. 41:254.

Vaitukaitis, J. L., J. B. Robbins, E. Nieschlag, and G. T. Ross. 1971. J. Clin. Endocr. 33:988.

Vaitukaitis, J. L., G. T. Ross, L. E. Reichert, and D. N. Ward. 1972. Endocrinology. 91:1337.

Van Vunakis, H., E. Wasserman, and L. Levine. 1972. J. Pharmacol. Exp. Ther. 180:514.

Van Weemen, B. K., and A. H. W. M. Schuurs. 1972. FEBS letters. 24:77.

Velick, S. F., C. W. Parker, and H. N. Eisen. 1960. Proc. Nat. Acad. Sci. USA. 46:1470.

Wainer, B. H., F. W. Fitch, J. Fried, and R. M. Rothberg. 1973. J. Immunol. 110:667.

Walsh, J. H., R. S. Yalow, and S. A. Berson. 1970. J. Infect. Dis. 121:550.

Warner, C., V. Schumaker, and F. Karush. 1970. Biochem. Biophys. Res. Commun. 38:125.

Weigle, W. O. 1964. Immunochemistry. 1:295.

Weintraub, B. D. 1970. Biochem. Biophys. Res. Commun. 39:83.

Werblin, T. P., and G. W. Siskind. 1972. Transplant. Rev. 8:104.

Whitney, P. L., and C. Tanford. 1965. Proc. Nat. Acad. Sci. USA. 53:524.

Wide, L. 1969. Acta Endocrinologica. Suppl. No. 142, p. 207.

Wide, L., H. Bennich, and S. G. O. Johansson. 1967. Lancet. 2:1105.

Wide, L., S. J. Nillius, C. Gemzell, and P. Roos. 1973. Acta Endocrinologica. Suppl. No. 174. p. 1.

Willams, C. A., and M. W. Chase (Eds.). 1967. Methods in immunology and immunochemistry. Vol. I. Academic Press, New York.

Wilzbach, K. E. 1957. J. Amer. Chem. Soc. 79:1013.

Wold, R. T., F. E. Young, E. M. Tan, and R. S. Farr. 1968. Science. 161:806.

Woodhead, J. S., G. M. Addison, and C. N. Hales. 1974. Brit. Med. Bull. 30:18.

Yalow, R. S., and S. A. Berson. 1960. J. Clin. Invest. 39:1157.

Yalow, R. S., and S. A. Berson. 1961. J. Clin. Invest. 40:2190.

Yalow, R. S., and S. A. Berson. 1969. *In* M. Margoulies (Ed.). Protein and polypeptide hormones. Excerpta Medica Fdn., Amsterdam. p. 37.

Yalow, R. S., and S. A. Berson. 1970*a*. Gastroenterology. 58.1.

Yalow, R. S., and S. A. Berson. 1970*b*. *In* J. W. McArthur, and T. Colton (Eds.). Statistics in endocrinology. MIT Press, Cambridge. p. 327.

Yalow, R. S., and S. A. Berson. 1971. *In* W. D. Odell, and W. H. Daughaday (Eds.). Principles of competitive protein-binding assays. J. B. Lippincott Co., Philadelphia. p. 374.

Yalow, R. S., S. M. Glick, J. Roth, and S. A. Berson. 1964. J. Clin. Endocrinol. Metab. 24:1219.

Young, J. D., and C. Y. Leon. 1970. Biochemistry. 9:2755.

Zull, J. E., and D. W. Repke. 1972. J. Biol. Chem. 247:2183.

Index

A

Absorbents, separating free from antibody-bound antigens with specific and nonspecific, 160-62

Absorption to eliminate cross reacting antibodies, 194-95

Administration of immunogens, 26-28

Affinity:
antibody, 111-38
  in antibody-hapten interactions, 111-12
  in antibody-protein interactions, 112-13
  cross-reactivity and role of hapten structure in, 39-40
  role of antigen valence in stabilization of immune complexes and, 113-16
  unequal competition of unlabeled antigen and antigen markers for antibodies, 116-17
  binding, 186

Amino acid sequences, role of primary, 45-46

Animal species, immunization of:
choosing species, 24
multiple species, 191

Animals, immunization of:
of multiple animals, 191
of partially tolerant animals, 194

Antibodies:
affinity of, 111-38

Antibodies (*cont.*)
affinity of (*cont.*)
  in antibody-hapten interactions, 111-12
  in antibody-protein interactions, 112-13
  cross reactivity and role of hapten structure in, 39-40
  role of antigen valence in stabilization of immune complexes and, 113-16
  unequal competition of unlabeled antigen and antigen markers for antibodies, 116-17
combining sites of, limitations in size of, 48-50
complementarity of, individual antiserum variation in, 37-38
cross-reacting, eliminated by absorption, 194-95
formation of, and reactivity to antigens, 52-59
heterogeneity of, 43-44, 117-20
  antibody fractionation and studies of heterogeneity by direct binding measurements, 119-20
  mathematical expression of, 117-19
quantitation of, 136
radioiodinated, 95-98
  immunologically complexed antibodies, 92-93
  used in fractionation of radioiodinated antigens, 95

229